CARDIOLOGY DEPT
BTC, CITY HOSPITAL

KT-428-342

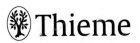

# Pocket Atlas of Echocardiography

Thomas Boehmeke, M.D.
Cardiology Practice
Gladbeck, Germany

Ralf Doliva, M.D.
Marienhospital Gelsenkirchen
Gelsenkirchen, Germany

444 illustrations

Thieme
Stuttgart · New York

*Library of Congress Cataloging-in-Publication Data* is available from the publisher.

This book is an authorized and revised translation of the German edition published and copyrighted 2004 by Georg Thieme Verlag, Stuttgart, Germany. Title of the German edition: Der Echo-Guide – Die kompakte Einführung in die Echokardiographie

Translator: Stephanie Kramer, B.A., Dipl. Trans., IoL, Berlin

Illustrators: Kirsten Haase and Benjamin Bode, Aachen

© 2006 Georg Thieme Verlag,
Rüdigerstrasse 14, 70469 Stuttgart, Germany
http://www.thieme.de
Thieme New York, 333 Seventh Avenue,
New York, NY 10001 USA
http://www.thieme.com

Typesetting by Satzpunkt Ewert, Bayreuth
Printed in Germany by Appl, Wemding
ISBN 3-13-141241-0 (GTV)
ISBN 1-58890-433-4 (TNY)

# Preface

Color Doppler echocardiography is the cornerstone of current diagnostic cardiology, facilitating targeted treatment by providing a wealth of functional data and information on morphologic changes. Learning how to use this fascinating tool, however, is complicated by the small size of the acoustic windows as well as the confusing number of imaging planes transecting the heart. The aim of this Echo-Guide is to make learning more accessible for the beginner.

This book would not have been possible in this form without the extensive support of Dr. Becker. We would also like to especially thank Kirsten Haase and Benjamin Bode (Aachen) for the excellent graphic design and Dr. Antje Schönpflug for her careful reading of the manuscript.

Thomas Böhmeke

# Contents

| Examination | 2 |
|---|---|
| Imaging and Patient Position | 2 |
| Parasternal Long-Axis View | 8 |
| Parasternal Short-Axis View | 14 |
| Apical Windows | 26 |
| Suprasternal Window | 36 |
| Subcostal Window | 40 |

| M-Mode and Doppler Echocardiography | 42 |
|---|---|
| M-Mode Echocardiography | 44 |
| Doppler Echocardiography | 48 |

| Cardiac Abnormalities | 76 |
|---|---|
| Valvular Heart Disease | 78 |
| Coronary Heart Disease | 132 |
| Cardiomyopathies | 150 |
| Prosthetic Valves | 164 |
| Carditis | 180 |
| Septal Defects | 194 |
| Hypertensive Heart Diseases | 204 |
| Intracardiac Masses | 212 |

# 1 Examination

Examination

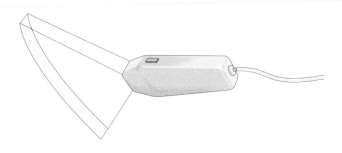

The phased-array transducers commonly used in echocardiography bear markings to indicate the scan plane.

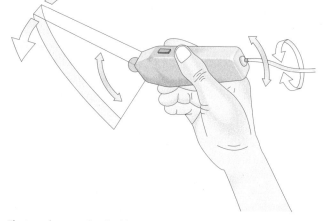

The transducer can be tilted (green arrows) and rotated (yellow arrows) to obtain various imaging planes.

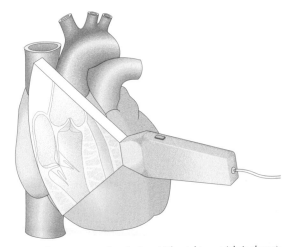

Ultrasound beam transecting the heart: The right ventricle is closest to the transducer, and the left ventricle and mitral valve are further behind.

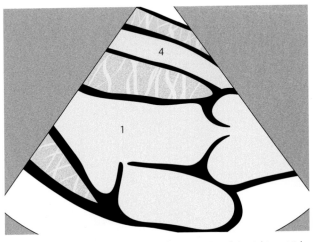

Corresponding monitor image: The projection of the right ventricle (located ventrally) is seen at the top.

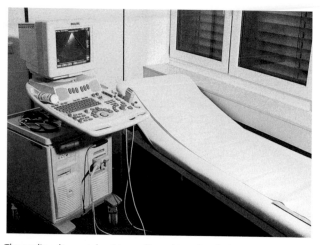

 The cardiac ultrasound unit is usually positioned to the left of the examining table.

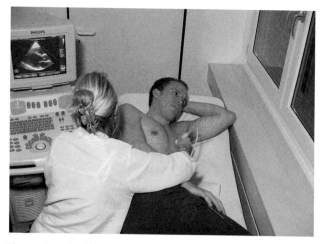

The examiner should be seated comfortably on a swivel stool.

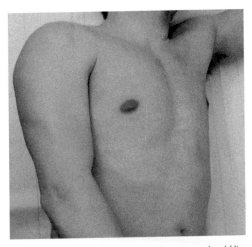

For the parasternal and apical windows, the patient should lie in the left lateral decubitus position.

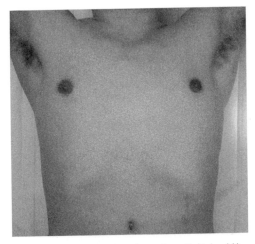

For the suprasternal and subcostal windows, the patient should lie in the supine position.

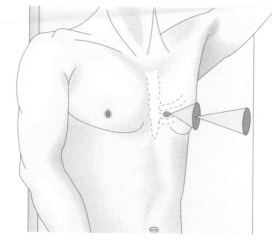

For the parasternal window, the patient lies in the left lateral position with the left arm behind his or her head. The acoustic window is situated in the fourth intercostal space just to the left of the sternum.

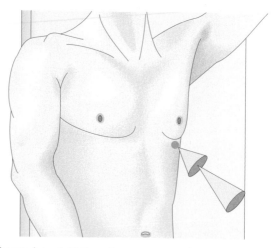

For the apical view (with the patient once again in the left lateral position) the beam is directed from the apical impulse.

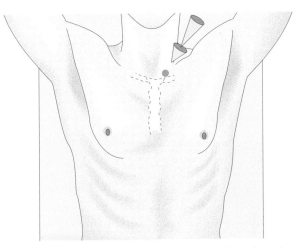

For the suprasternal window the patient lies in the supine position. The beam is directed from the suprasternal notch toward the aortic arch.

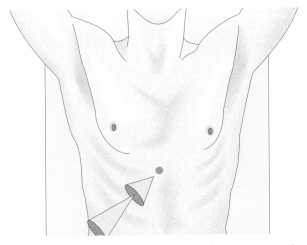

For the subcostal window (with the patient once again in the supine position), the heart is imaged from below.

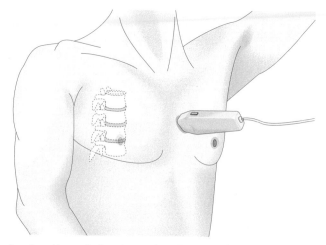

Parasternal long-axis view: Coming from the fourth intercostal space just left of the sternum (the window/orifice allowing free access past the lung is merely the size of a postage stamp) the transducer is aimed perpendicularly toward the spine.

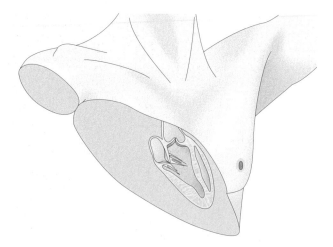

The plane of the beam runs between the axilla and lower left costal arch.

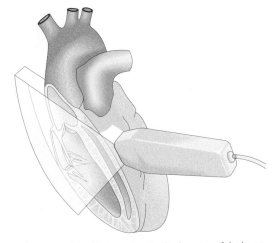

The ultrasound plane displays a longitudinal section of the heart from the tip of the ventricle to the aorta.

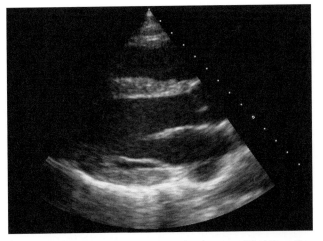

The right ventricle is displayed at the top and the left cardiac structures below.

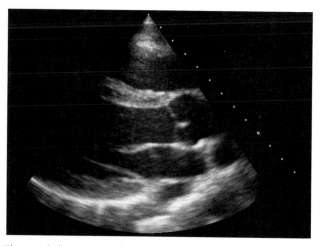

The aortic bulb seen just at the right of the center of the image can be used to check orientation; beneath it is the mitral valve and to its left is the left ventricle.

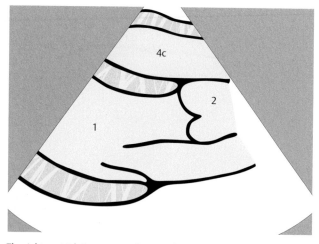

The right ventricle is seen near the transducer. The left ventricle is on the left and the aortic valve is just at the right of the center.

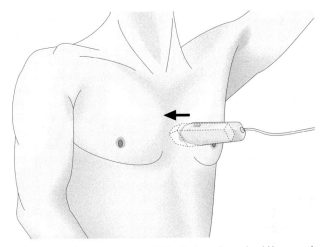

If no cardiac structures are visible, the transducer should be moved directly toward the sternum ...

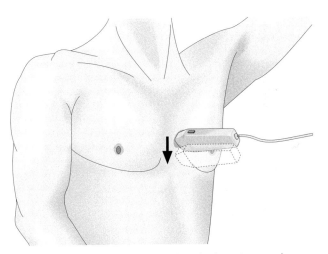

... or the beam should be directed through a lower intercostal space.

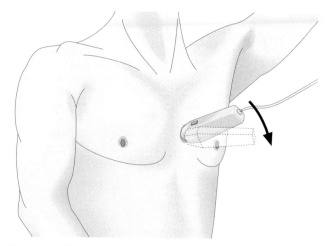

If too much of the left ventricle is visible, the imaging plane should be tilted craniad, i.e., the transducer cord moved toward the left iliac crest.

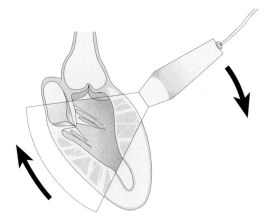

Imaging plane tilted too far caudad: Only the left ventricle is visible.

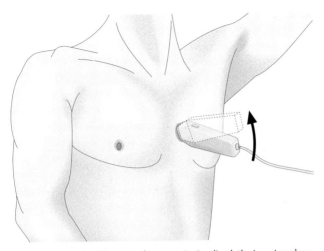

If too much of the ascending aorta is visualized, the imaging plane can be tilted caudad, i.e., the transducer cord moved toward the right shoulder.

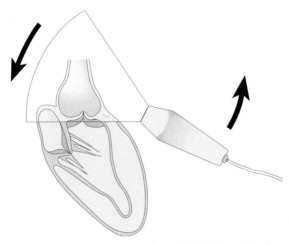

Imaging plane tilted too far craniad: Predominating view of ascending aorta.

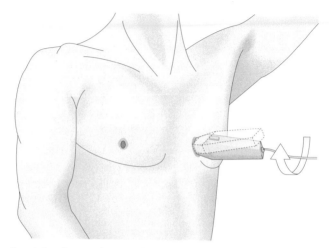

On rotating the transducer 90° clockwise, the heart is imaged in the parasternal short-axis view.

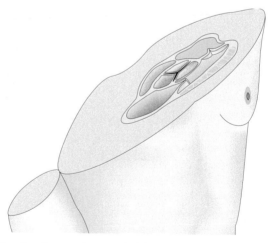

The imaging plane runs between the left axilla and right costal arch.

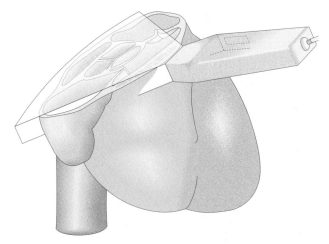

A cross-section of the heart is visible at the level of the aortic valve. ◀

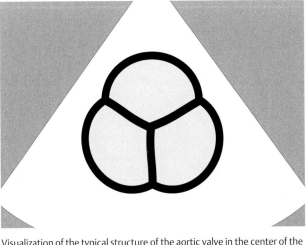

Visualization of the typical structure of the aortic valve in the center of the image helps to check orientation. ◀

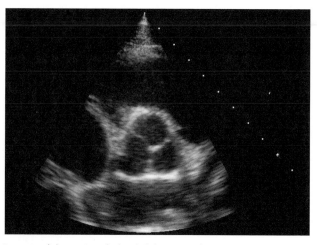

Parasternal short axis at the level of the aortic valve.

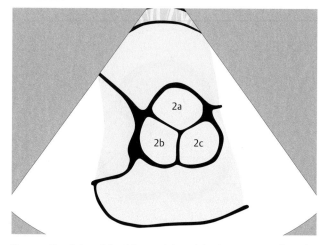

Cross-sectional view of the right ventricle and the three crescent-shaped leaflets of the aortic valve.

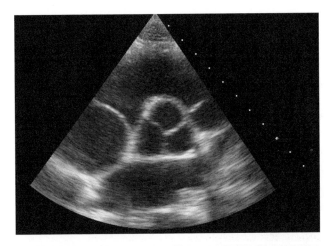

Short-axis parasternal view of the aortic valve in the center surrounded by adjacent right cardiac structures.

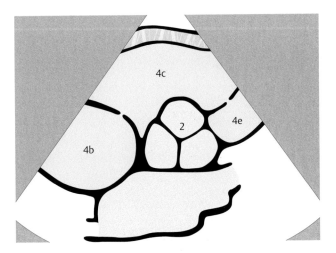

Tricuspid and pulmonary valves in the parasternal short-axis view.

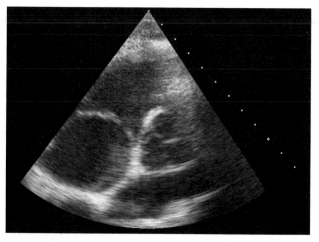

 If the transducer is not rotated exactly within the parasternal window, lung tissue can often be superimposed.

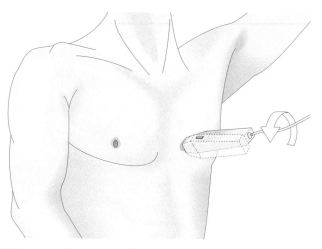

If orientation is lost, return to the parasternal long-axis view and begin again from the start.

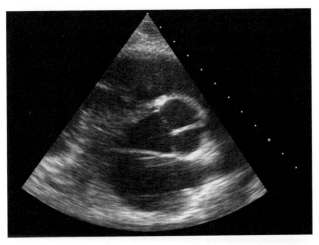

A suboptimal imaging plane can result in a slanted transection of the aortic leaflets.

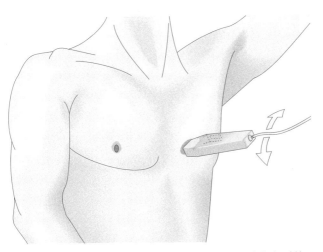

Rotating the transducer a few degrees to the right or left should be sufficient to correct the image.

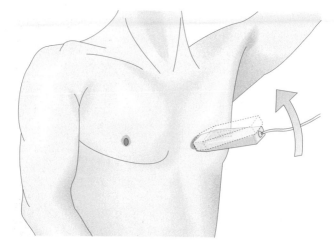

 Slightly tilting the plane of the ultrasound beam caudad (transducer cord toward the right shoulder) allows a cross-sectional view of the mitral valve.

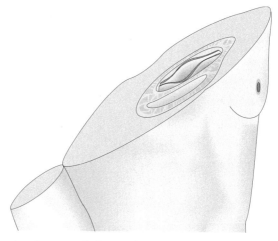

The valve edges are easily distinguished.

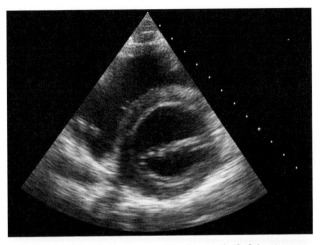

The motion of the mitral valve resembles the mouth of a fish as it opens.

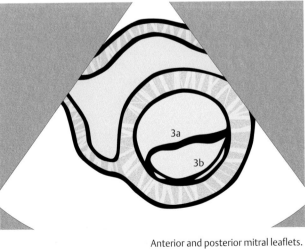

3a

3b

Anterior and posterior mitral leaflets.

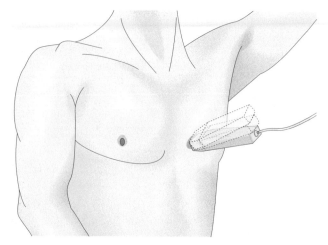

The chordae tendinae can be imaged by tilting the plane of the ultrasound beam caudad.

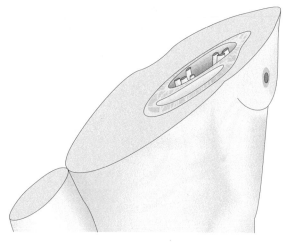

The beam intersects the chordae tendinae in a cross-wise fashion.

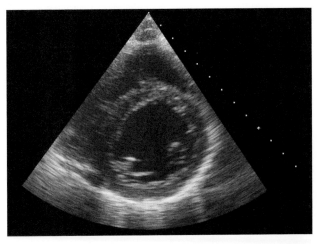

If correctly intersected by the beam, the left ventricle appears
as a perfect circle.

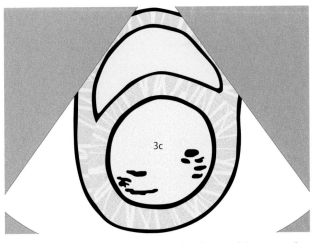

In this plane a good evaluation of the contractility
of the left ventricular segments near the base can be carried out.

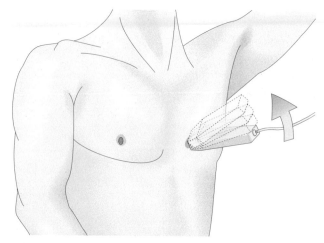

By further tilting the ultrasound plane caudad, a cross-sectional view of the papillary muscles is obtained.

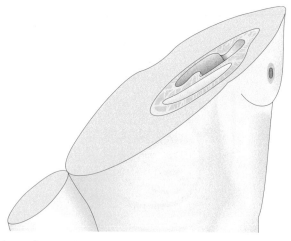

The papillary muscles and the center of the left ventricle are transected cross-wise by the beam.

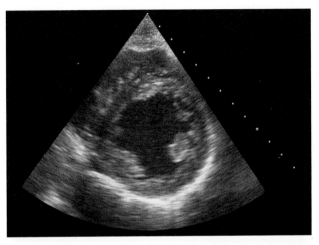

Note the round appearance of the left ventricle also in this plane.

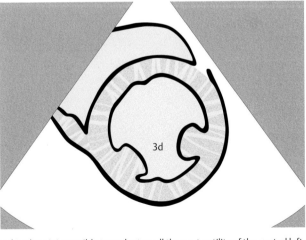

In this plane it is possible to evaluate well the contractility of the central left ventricular segments.

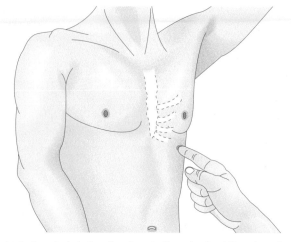

To obtain the apical window, first the apical impulse should be palpated.

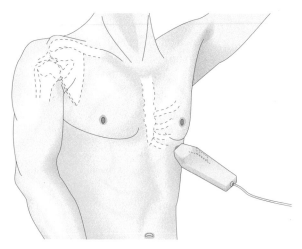

The transducer is placed on the apical impulse and is aimed toward the right shoulder blade.

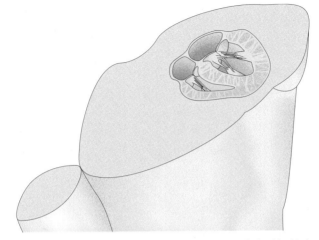

The first imaging plane runs between the left shoulder blade and right costal arch, the transducer marking directed toward the left shoulder blade. ◀

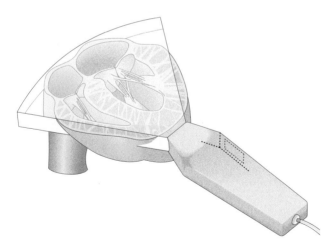

Both ventricles and atria can be visualized from the apex of the heart. ◀

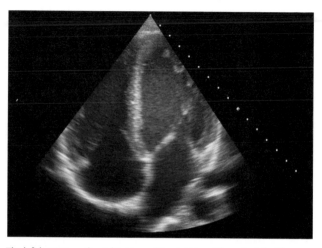

The left heart is on the right side and the right heart is on the left side of the image.

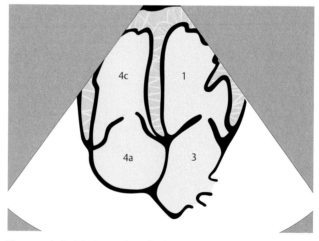

The upper half of the image shows both ventricles, beneath them are the right and left atria. The ventricles and atria are separated by the mitral and tricuspid valves.

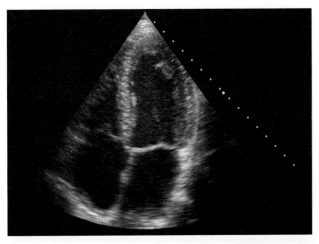

The right heart is usually visualized in less detail than the left.

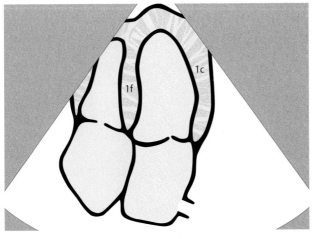

The lateral wall of the left ventricle is on the right; the septal wall is in the center.

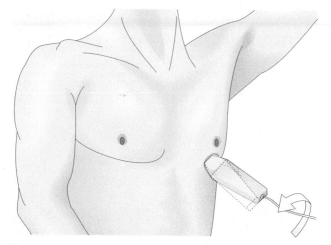

The apical two-chamber view is obtained by rotating the transducer 60° counterclockwise.

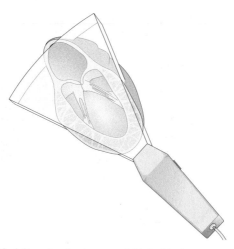

Only the left cardiac structures are visible in this plane.

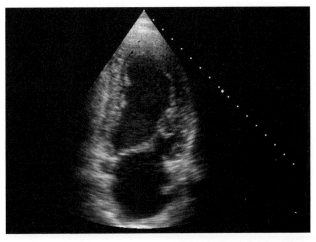

The papillary muscle often appears prominently in this plane. ◄

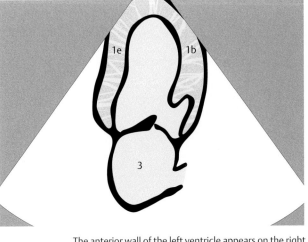

The anterior wall of the left ventricle appears on the right and the inferior wall on the left side. ◄

Examination

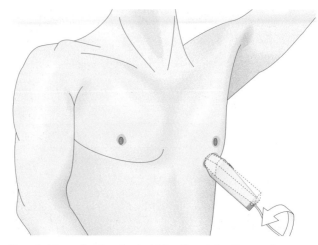

The apical three-chamber view is obtained by rotating the transducer 60° further counterclockwise.

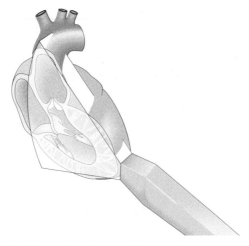

The aortic bulb is now imaged as an additional cardiac structure.

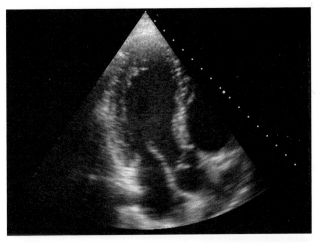

Left ventricular inflow and outflow can be evaluated well in this plane.

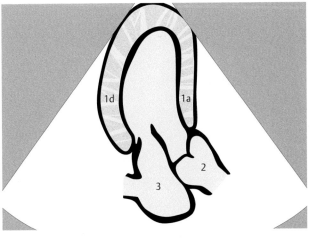

The anteroseptal wall of the left ventricle is displayed on the right
and the posterior wall on the left side of the image.

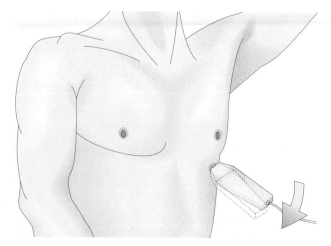

To image the "fifth chamber" the transducer is tilted slightly caudad from the four-chamber view.

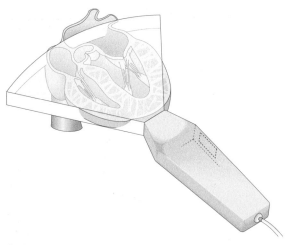

The five-chamber view shows both the atria and the ventricles, as well as the aortic bulb in between representing the "fifth chamber."

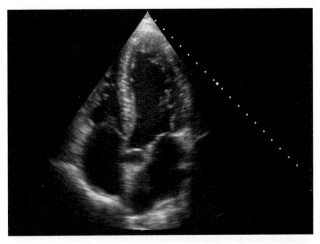

Left ventricular outflow across the aortic valve can be evaluated well here.

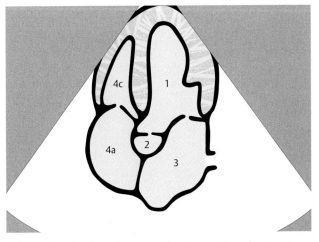

The five-chamber view offers an overview of the main cardiac structures.

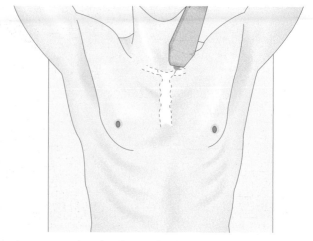

For the suprasternal window the transducer is placed in the suprasternal notch or just above the upper left sternal border.

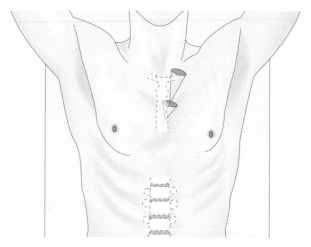

The beam is directed toward the lumbar vertebrae.

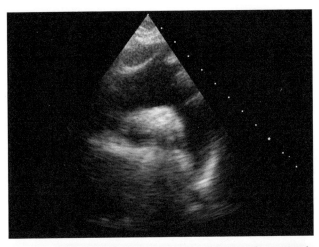

Complete visualization of the ascending aorta, the aortic arch and the descending aorta is usually only possible in young patients.

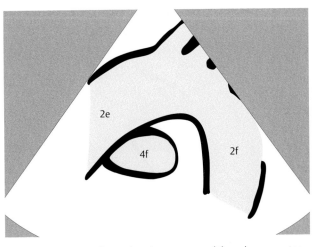

The aortic arch curves around the pulmonary artery.

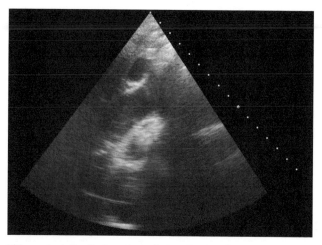

Tilting and rotating the transducer displays the ascending aorta and aortic arch.

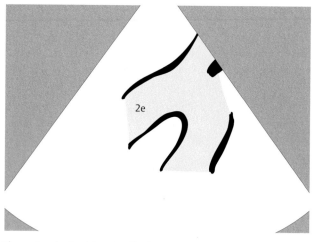

2e

The aortic valve is seldom visualized.

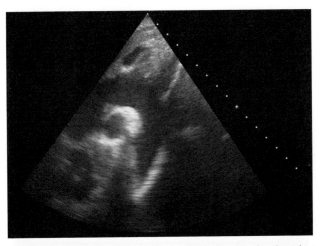

The supra-aortic arteries typically run diagonally upward to the right.

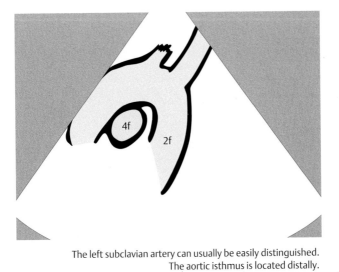

The left subclavian artery can usually be easily distinguished.
The aortic isthmus is located distally.

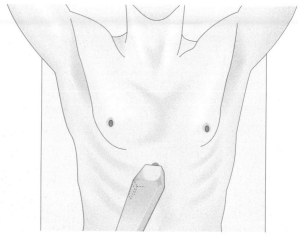

For the subcostal window the transducer is placed directly beneath the xyphoid or in the left subcostal area.

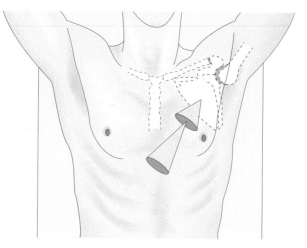

The ultrasound beam is aimed toward the left shoulder.

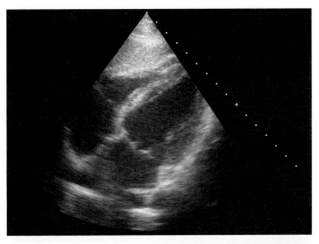

Four-chamber view tilted to the right.

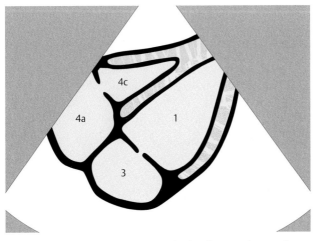

The right atrium and right ventricle are displayed nearest the transducer.

# 2 M-Mode and Doppler Echocardiography

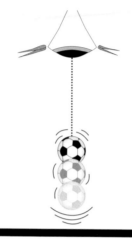

M-mode echocardiography provides unidimensional imaging of moving objects over time. Only the top point of the soccer ball is detected ...

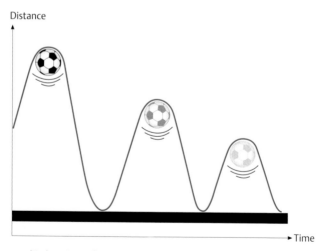

... and its location is shown over time.

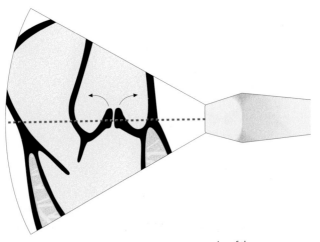

M-mode records the characteristic echo of the noncoronary and left coronary aortic leaflets, behind which is the left atrium (parasternal window).

Open valve    Closed valve

Left atrium

Characteristic parallelogram of the aortic valve opening in systole. In diastole the valve edges appear as a highly reflective line.

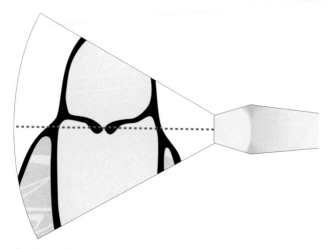

The ultrasound beam traces the typical biphasic pattern of mitral valve opening motion (first wave: ventricle relaxation, second wave: atrial contraction).

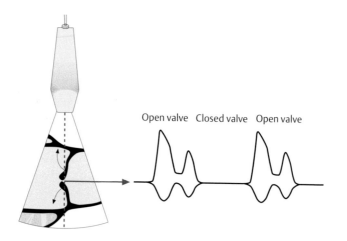

Open valve    Closed valve    Open valve

The monitor shows the M-shaped pattern of movement of the anterior mitral leaflet above and the small W-shaped pattern of the posterior leaflet below.

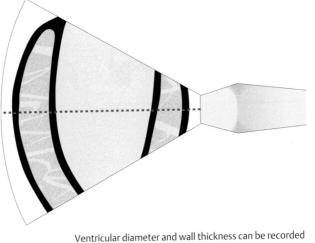

Ventricular diameter and wall thickness can be recorded in the parasternal view.

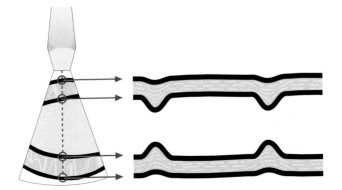

Typical thickening and inward motion of the myocardium can be seen in systole.

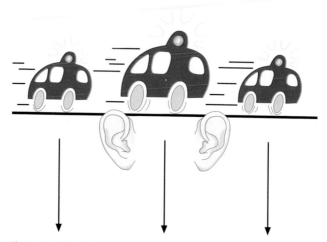

The Doppler effect describes the change in frequency of a moving source of sound. The sound of an approaching ambulance is perceived to be higher pitched ...

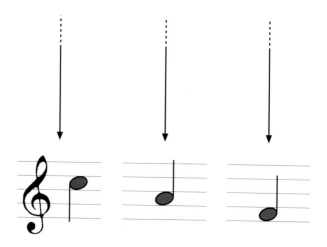

... than the sound of one driving away. Velocity can be calculated based on the frequency shift.

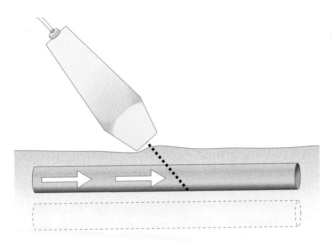

Using the Doppler principle, it is possible to image blood flow not only in terms of velocity ...

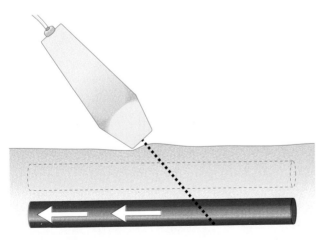

... but also in terms of flow direction.

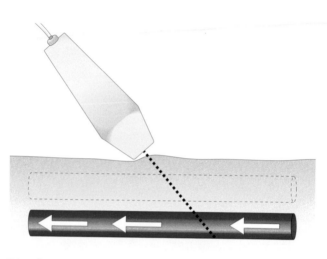

When the transducer is positioned at the angle shown in the diagram, the direction of blood flow is toward the transducer head.

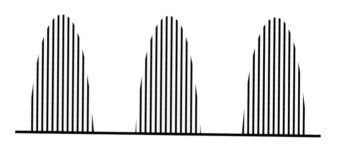

Motion toward the transducer is displayed above the zero baseline on the monitor.

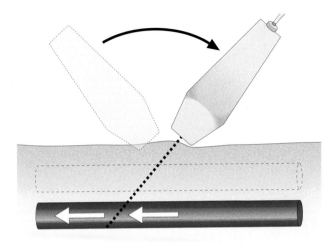

If the transducer is tilted in the opposite direction, the Doppler signal records blood flow moving away from it.

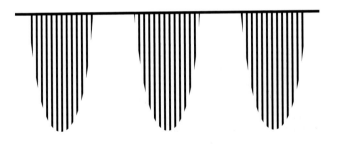

Motion away from the transducer is shown below the zero baseline on the monitor.

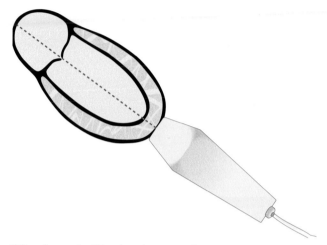

 CW mode records all Doppler pulses in a unidimensional ultrasound beam.

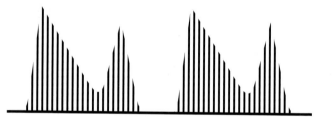

 CW Doppler recording of transmitral flow: Flow into the left ventricle is toward the transducer and therefore displayed above the zero baseline.

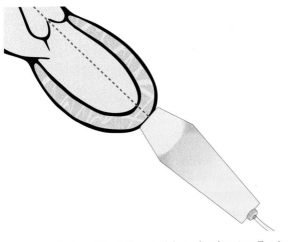

Aortic outflow in the apical three-chamber view: Flow is away from the transducer ...

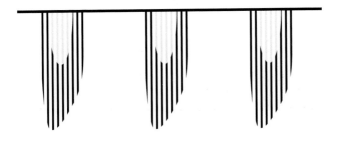

... and thus displayed below the zero baseline.

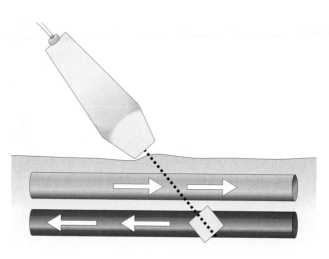

Pulsed-wave Doppler mode enables imaging of velocities within a chosen window.

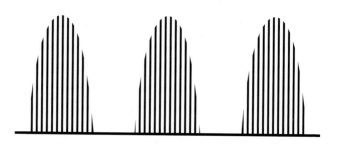

As in the CW mode, flow toward the transducer is shown above the zero baseline.

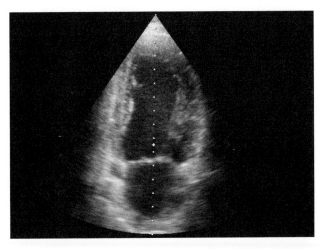

PW mode is suitable for evaluating transmitral inflow in the apical two-chamber view.

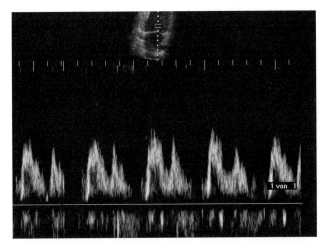

The Doppler spectrum shows the typical M-shaped profile of transmitral inflow.

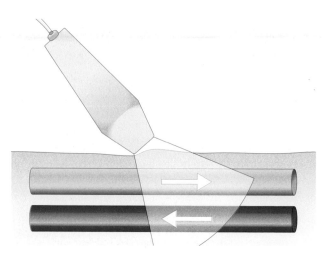

Color Doppler imaging depicts all flows in a chosen sector.

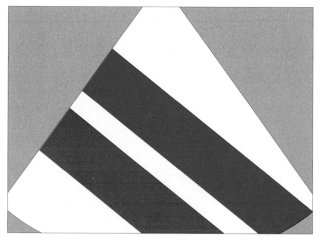

Flow toward the transducer is displayed in red; flow away from the transducer is displayed in blue.

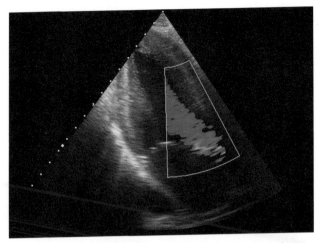

All flows within a chosen segment of the two-dimensional image are analyzed and displayed in color.

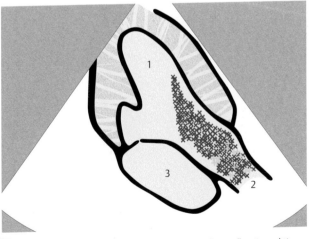

Color Doppler imaging showing left ventricular outflow in real time; because flow is away from the transducer it is blue in color.

At higher velocities (usually greater than 1 m/s) flow is displayed in yellow-white; flow direction is not differentiated.

Increased flow velocity in a narrowed vessel segment displayed in yellow-white.

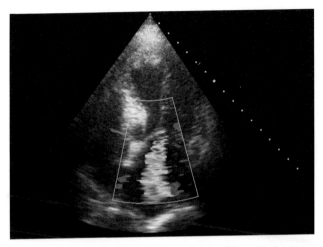

Example of mitral insufficiency in an apical four-chamber view:
Retrograde flow appears across the insufficient valve in systole.

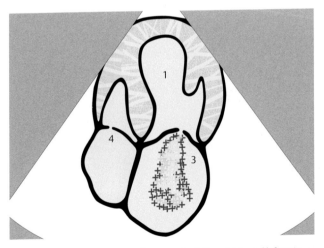

Due to the difference in pressure between the left ventricle and left atrium,
velocity is greater than 4 m/s and thus displayed in yellow-white.

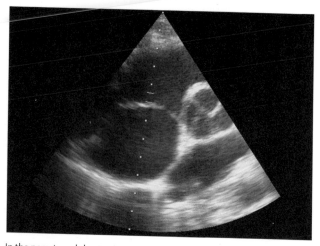

In the parasternal short-axis view, PW Doppler can be positioned across the tricuspid valve.

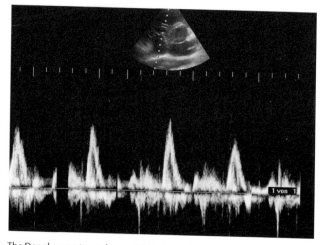

The Doppler spectrum shows a biphasic, M-shaped inflow profile.

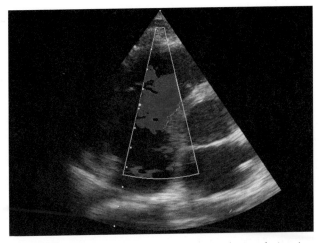

Tricuspid inflow can also be displayed using color Doppler imaging (parasternal short-axis view).

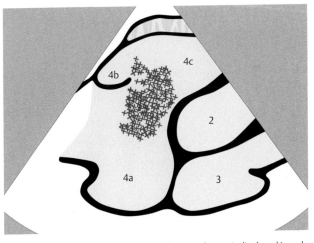

Inflow in the right ventricle—toward the transducer—is displayed in red.

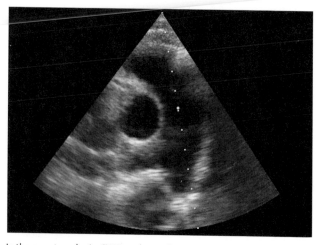

In the parasternal axis, CW Doppler can be positioned in the pulmonary artery.

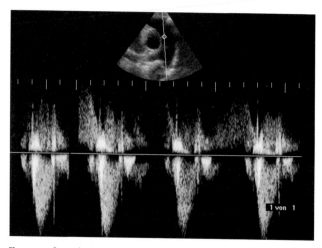

Flow away from the transducer appears V-shaped, below the zero baseline.

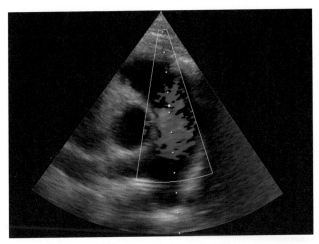

Pulmonary outflow into the bifurcation of the pulmonary arteries
can usually be fully imaged only in young patients.

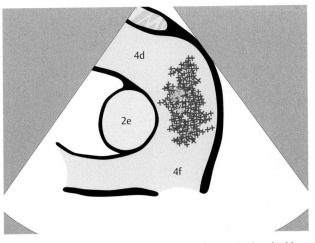

Flow away from the transducer is displayed in blue.

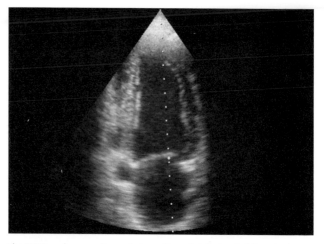

The PW Doppler recording gate is positioned at the level of the mitral valve edges.

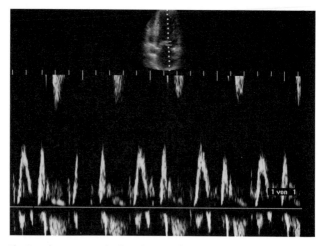

The Doppler spectrum displays the typical M-shaped profile of mitral inflow.

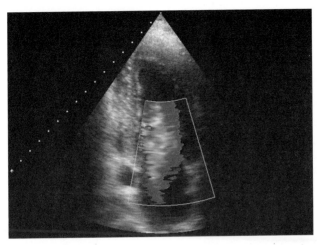

Color Doppler displays the broad mitral inflow in the left ventricle. ◀

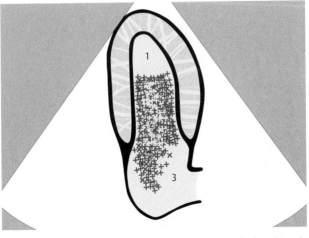

Flow toward the transducer is displayed in red. ◀

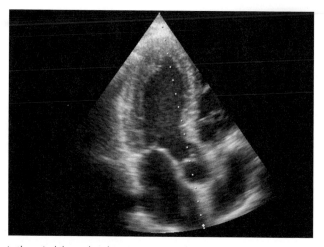

In the apical three-chamber view, CW Doppler can be positioned in the left ventricular outflow tract.

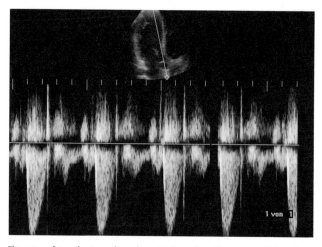

Flow away from the transducer has a V-shaped profile, comparable with that across the pulmonary valve.

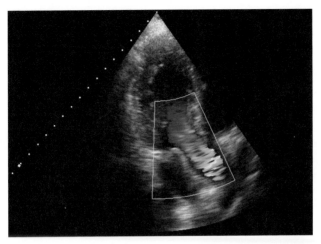

Color Doppler imaging shows outflow from the ventricle up into the ascending aorta.

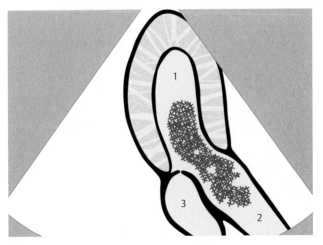

Isolated increases in flow velocity, displayed in yellow, are not necessarily a sign of clinically relevant aortic stenosis.

M- Mode and Doppler Echocardiography

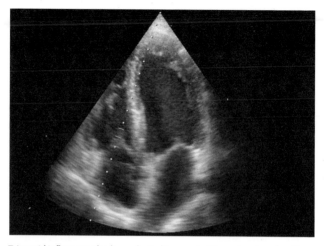

Tricuspid inflow can also be evaluated in an apical four-chamber view if it is not readily visible in the parasternal view.

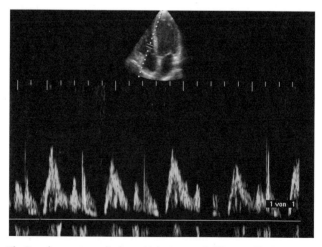

The Doppler spectrum displays a biphasic recorded flow profile above the zero baseline.

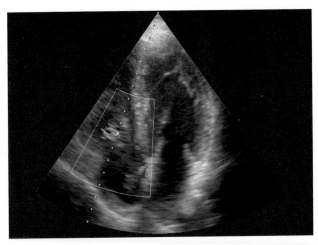

In Doppler color imaging, right cardiac flows appear less intense than left cardiac flows.

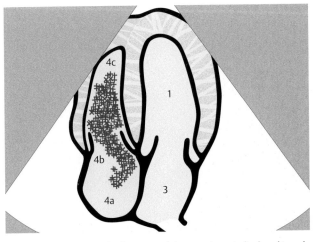

Tricuspid inflow toward the transducer is displayed in red.

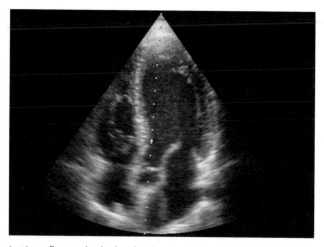

Aortic outflow can be displayed in the apical three-chamber or five-chamber view.

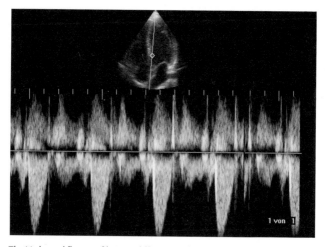

The V-shaped flow profile is no different to the Doppler spectrum seen in the three-chamber view.

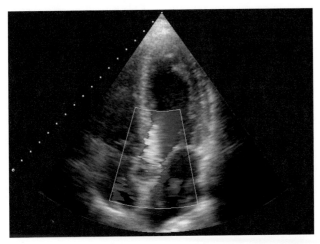

The imaged sector shows blue-color flow in the left ventricular
outflow tract. ◀

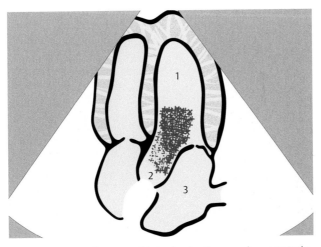

It is usually not possible to visualize the ascending aorta in the
five-chamber view; here the three-chamber view is more suitable. ◀

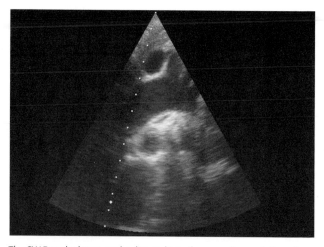

The CW Doppler beam can be directed into the ascending aorta from the suprasternal window.

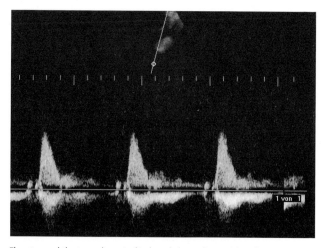

Flow toward the transducer is displayed above the zero baseline.

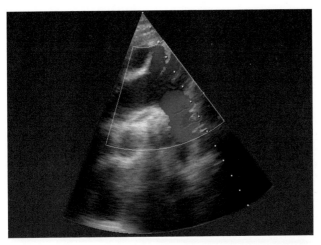

Color Doppler imaging of the aortic arch can be used to evaluate subclavian stenosis or aortic isthmus stenosis.

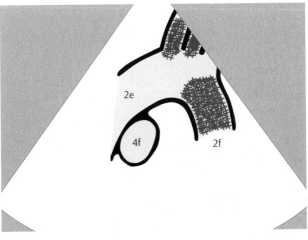

Flow in the descending aorta away from the transducer is displayed in blue; flow in the supra-aortic arteries is displayed in red.

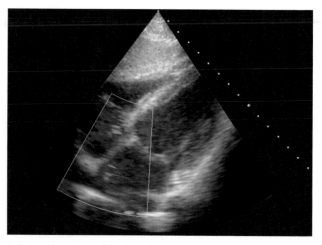

Color Doppler imaging from the subcostal window usually allows better depiction of flow conditions in the atria than in the apical four-chamber view.

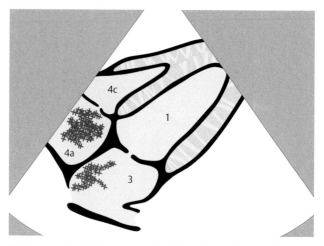

Furthermore, the atrial septum can be distinguished well in this plane.

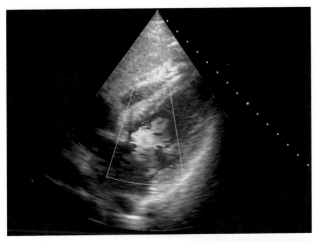

Transmitral inflow is displayed in red.     ◀

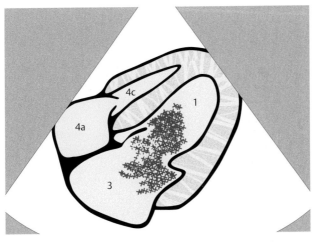

Isolated increases in flow velocity, displayed in yellow, can also occur in a normal mitral valve.     ◀

# 3 Cardiac Abnormalities

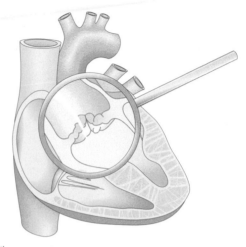

Calcified semilunar cusps in aortic stenosis.

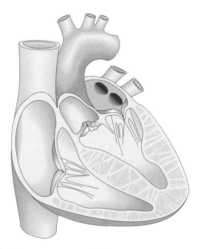

Pressure overload causes concentric left ventricular hypertrophy.

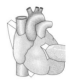

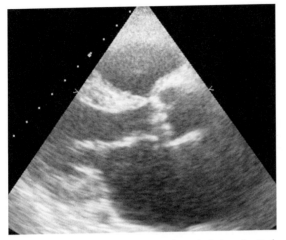

The parasternal short-axis view is particularly well-suited for visualizing decreased opening motion ...

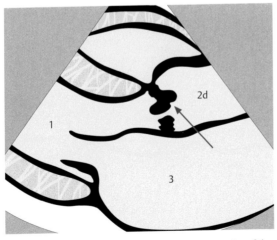

... although separation does not permit estimation of the degree of stenosis.

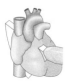

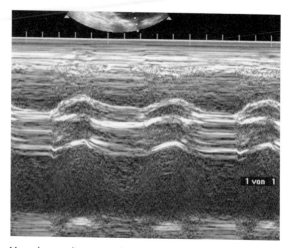

M-mode recording across the aortic valve shows echodense, bandlike reflections of the calcified valve apparatus with reduced opening motion.

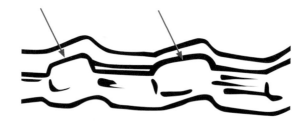

Separation cannot be thoroughly displayed and provides no indication of degree of stenosis.

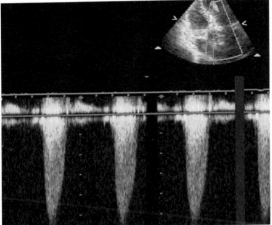
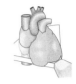

The accelerated outflow across the aortic valve is represented in the continuous-wave (CW) Doppler mode by a V-shaped flow profile with increased velocities.

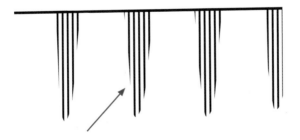

The recorded velocities (preferably including stroke volume) are used for quantification purposes.

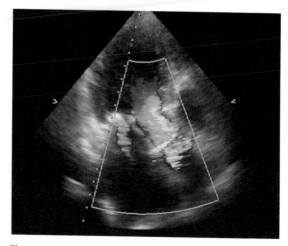

The stenotic aortic valve causes an increase in flow velocity ...

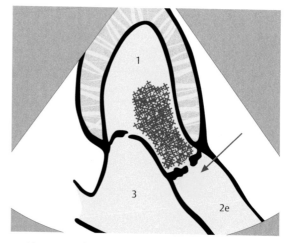

... with corresponding color change above the valve.

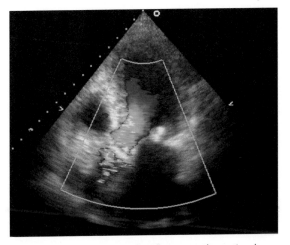

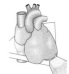

Increased outflow across the aortic valve ...

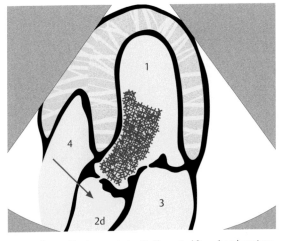

... can be readily demonstrated in the apical five-chamber view.

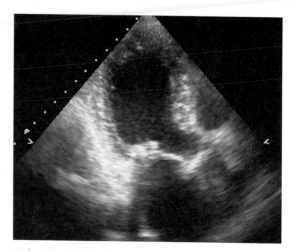

Moderately calcified valves in medium-grade aortic stenosis.

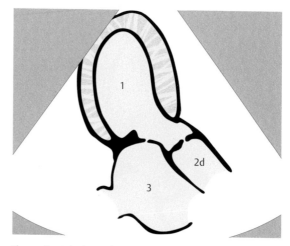

The moderately elevated pressure gradient has not caused hypertrophy of the left ventricle.

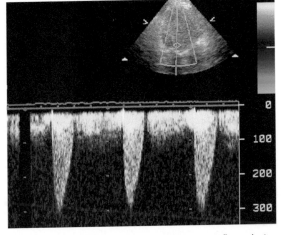

CW Doppler mode displays a moderate rise in flow velocity up to approximately 3 m/s.

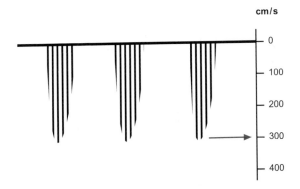

Computer-assisted conversion yields a maximum gradient of 36 mmHg.

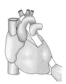

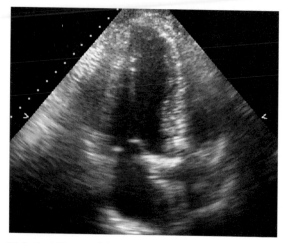

Marked calcification of the aortic valve.

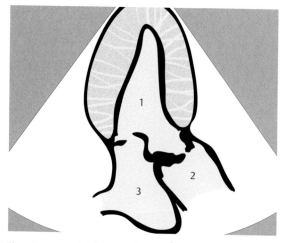

There is concentric left ventricular hypertrophy.

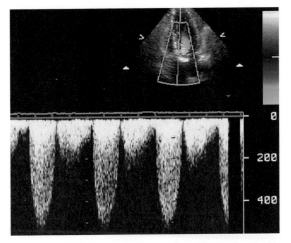

CW Doppler demonstrating a rise in flow velocity up to 5 m/s, corresponding to a maximum gradient of 100 mmHg.

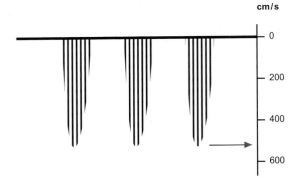

Patience and time are necessary to obtain a usable CW analysis of transaortic flow.

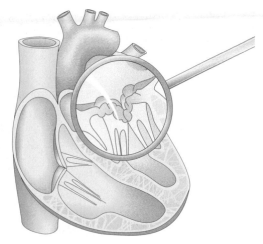

Calcified mitral valve in mitral stenosis.

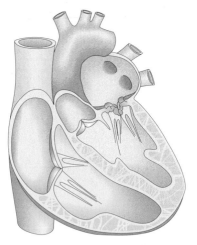

Dilatation of the left atrium and right heart as a result of pressure overload.

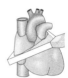

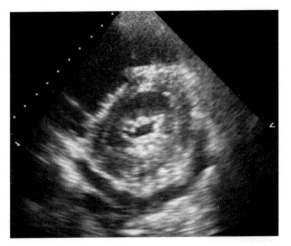

In the parasternal short-axis view, the remaining mitral valve orifice area can be seen directly …

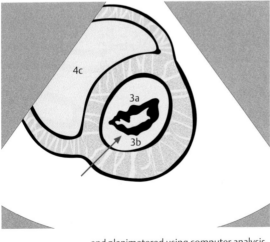

… and planimetered using computer analysis.
Under good visualization, this value can be used for quantification.

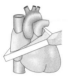

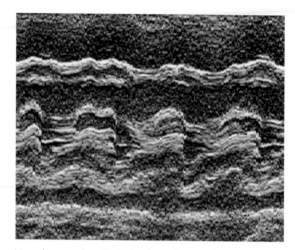

M-mode across the mitral valve shows decreased opening motion of both leaflets.

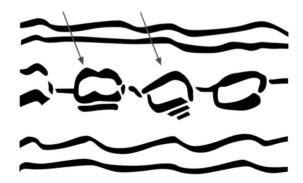

Limited opening motion is not a valid parameter for estimating degree of severity.

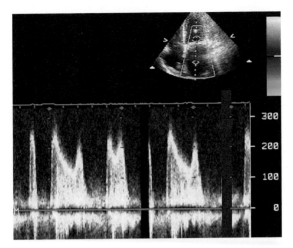

CW Doppler recording showing increased transmitral velocity
as well as a flat decline in transmitral inflow.

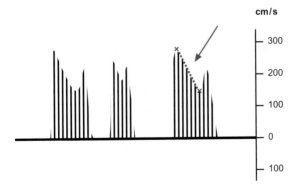

Computer-assisted measurement of diastolic pressure gradient
is used for quantification (so-called pressure half-time).

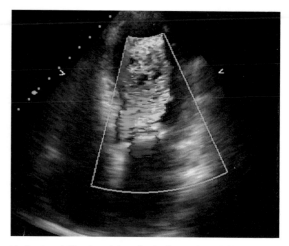

Moderate calcification of the valve leaflets and atrial dilatation.

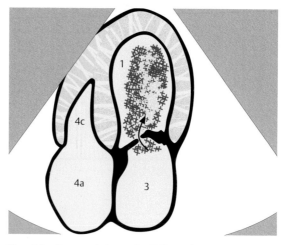

The minimal increase in transmitral inflow velocity causes a circumscribed color change.

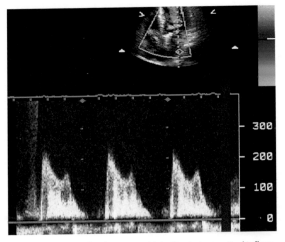

CW Doppler shows a rapid decline in transmitral inflow.

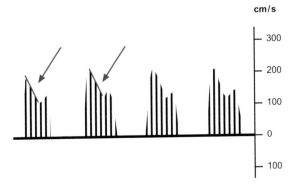

cm/s

Computer-assisted quantification yields a functional valve orifice area of >2 cm².

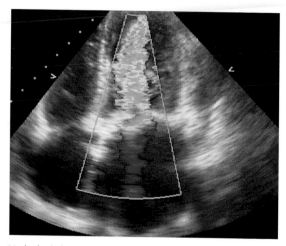

Marked calcification of the mitral valves as well as a considerably dilated left atrium can be seen.

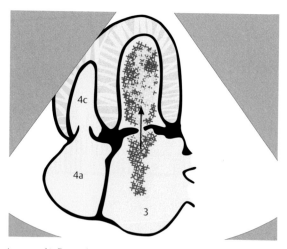

Increased inflow velocity across the stenotic valve appears like a candle flame in the image.

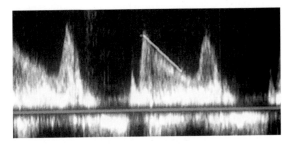

CW Doppler imaging shows a slow decrease in transmitral inflow velocity.

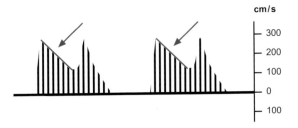

Analysis of the slope velocity yields a valve orifice area of 1.0 cm².

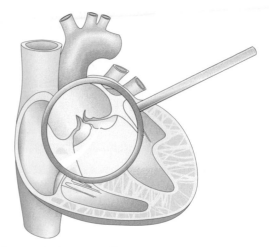

Aortic valve degeneration in aortic insufficiency.

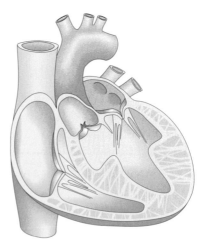

Volume overload results in eccentric left ventricular hypertrophy.

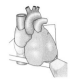

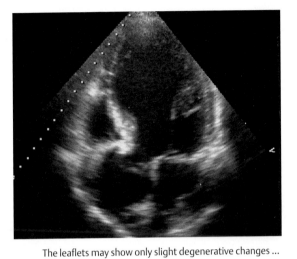

The leaflets may show only slight degenerative changes ...

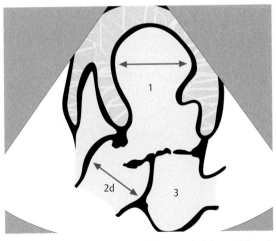

... whereas in more severe aortic insufficiency the left ventricle and ascending aorta are dilated.

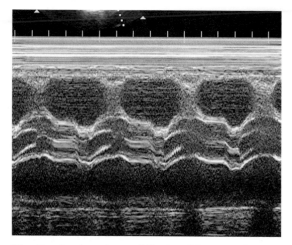

Often there is only moderate calcification of the aortic valve leaflets with normal opening motion in M-mode.

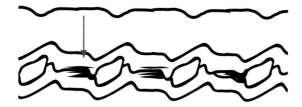

Leakage through the aortic valve leaflets in diastole cannot be imaged in M-mode.

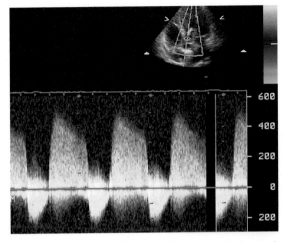

The alignment of retrograde flow signals is performed in the apical windows and demonstrates the typical steplike signal produced by aortic insufficiency.

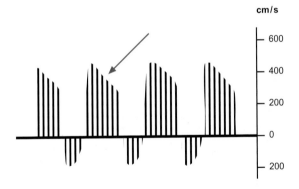

Evidence of a regurgitant jet can be analyzed only qualitatively in CW Doppler; quantification is conducted with color Doppler imaging.

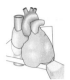

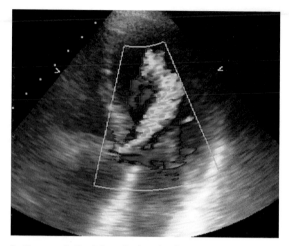

Aortic regurgitation is best displayed in the apical windows.

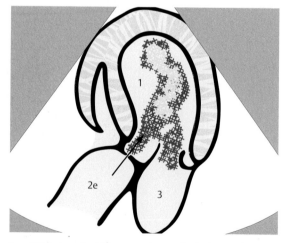

Even if the regurgitant jet appears impressive in the apical window ...

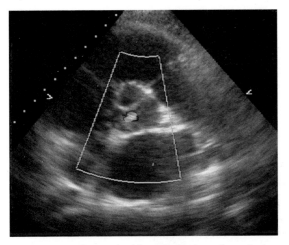

... quantification should nonetheless be performed using cross-sectional imaging in the parasternal short-axis view ...

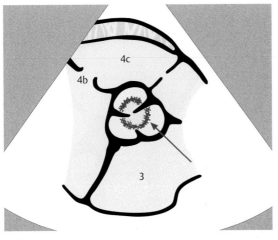

... and it should be evaluated in relation to the cross-section of the left ventricular outflow tract.

Cardiac Abnormalities

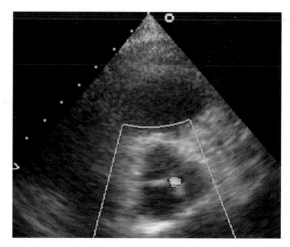

Color Doppler imaging can display the regurgitation orifice in the parasternal short-axis view.

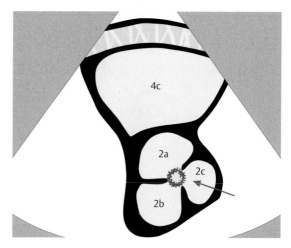

In mild aortic insufficiency, the regurgitation orifice is small compared with a cross-sectional view of the infundibulum.

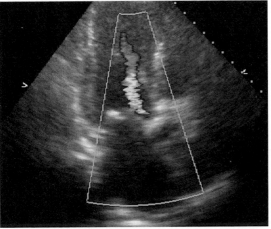

From an apical view, only a narrow regurgitant jet can be seen.

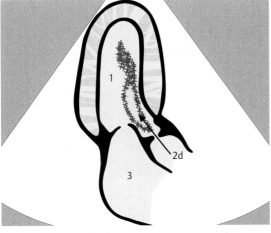

Aortic regurgitation can restrict the opening motion
of the anterior mitral leaflet.

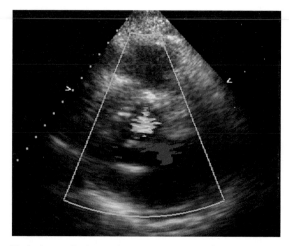

Marked regurgitation can be seen in a parasternal view ...

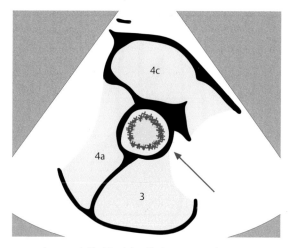

... covering over half of the infundibular cross-section.

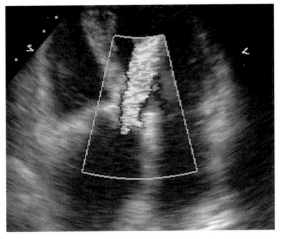

Correspondingly there is a wide regurgitant jet in the apical view.

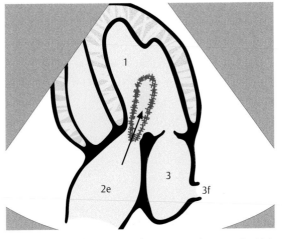

Under increased intraventricular pressures, the regurgitant jet does not reach the ventricular apex.

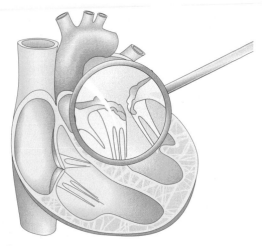

Degenerative changes in a mitral valve in mitral insufficiency.

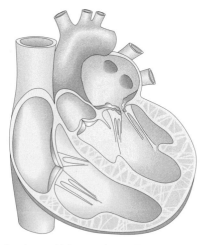

Dilatation of left atrium and left ventricle as well as right heart dilatation due to volume overload.

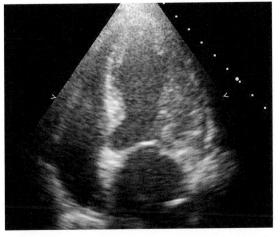

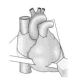

Dilatation of the left atrium is visible in the foreground.

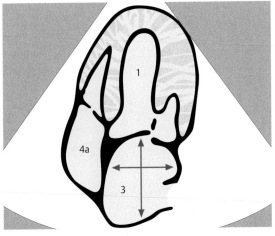

Dilatation of the right heart can also occur in higher-grade mitral insufficiency.

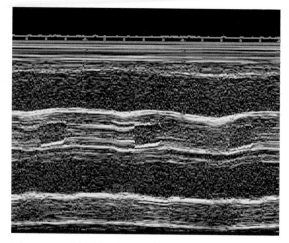

Enlargement of the left atrium can be demonstrated
in an M-mode recording of the aorta.

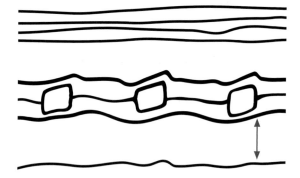

Atrial size should be measured at end systole.

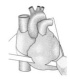

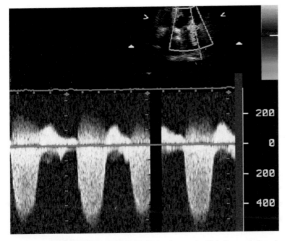

CW Doppler imaging displays the typical U-shaped signal of a regurgitant jet.

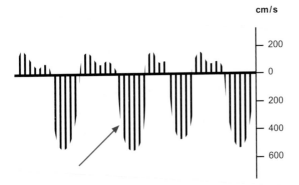

Velocity is not an indicator of the degree of insufficiency.

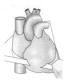

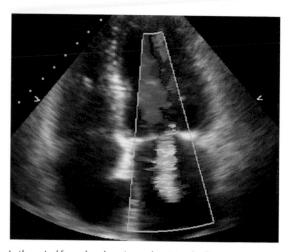

In the apical four-chamber view only minimal reflux across the mitral valve can be seen.

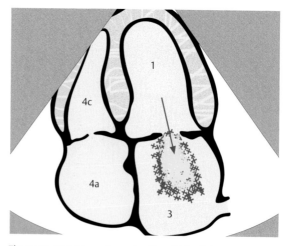

The regurgitant jet nearly reaches the middle of the atrium.

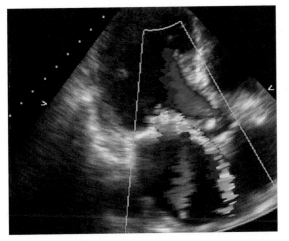

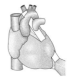

The insufficiency should be imaged in several planes
as it may be eccentric.

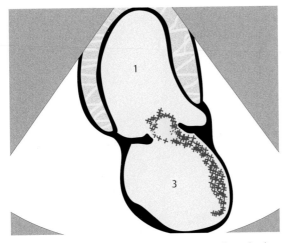

Imaging the insufficiency in one plane only can lead to
overestimation or underestimation of its severity.

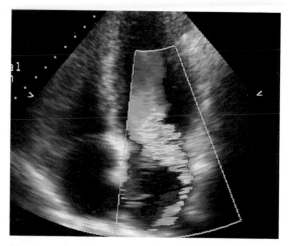

A pronounced regurgitant jet in the left atrium.

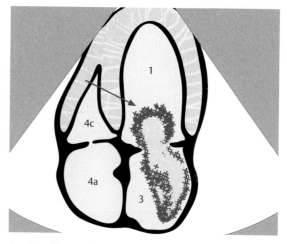

As a sign of increased intraventricular flow toward the valve leakage, a change in color is seen before the mitral valve.

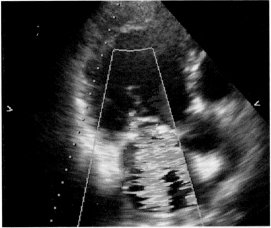

Regurgitation into the left atrium is also predominant in the apical two-chamber view.

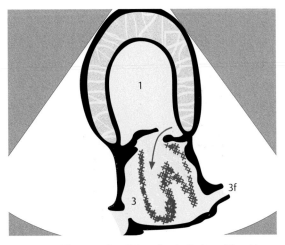

The regurgitant jet reaches to the top of the atrium.

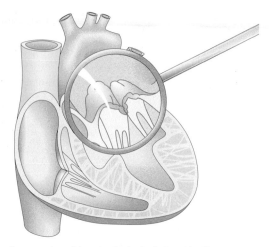

Myxomatous degeneration of the mitral valve is distinguished by elongated, thickened leaflets which prolapse into the atrium.

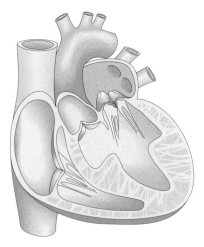

Depending on the extent of concomitant mitral insufficiency, there can be dilatation of the left atrium.

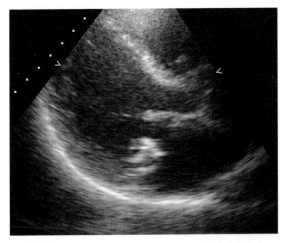
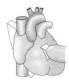

The thickened leaflets can calcify, making them more difficult to distinguish from vegetations related to endocarditis.

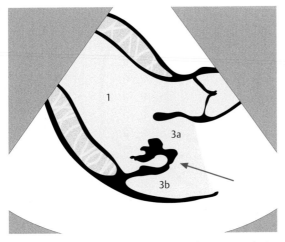

Diagnosis of mitral valve prolapse is made in the parasternal axis; apical windows often reveal (false-positive) prolapse.

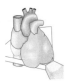

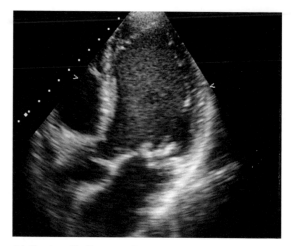

Calcification of leaflet areas affected by myxomatous degeneration can be imaged in the apical windows.

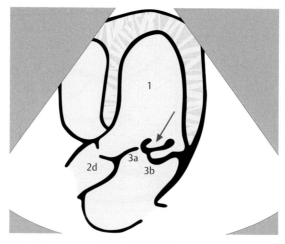

Elongation can cause folding of the leaflets.

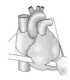

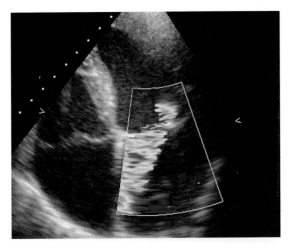

Prolapse of the posterior mitral leaflet typically leads to an eccentric regurgitant jet.

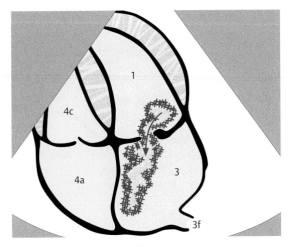

Accelerated flow toward the valve leakage created in the ventricle implicates a higher degree of mitral insufficiency (flow convergence zone).

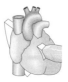

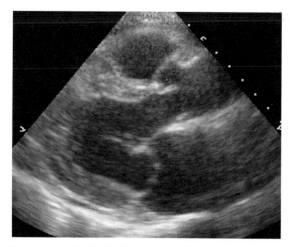

The posterior mitral leaflet is elongated and "doming" into the left atrium.

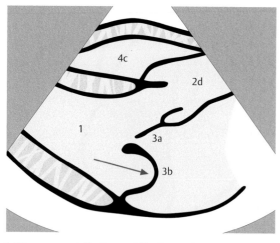

In this case, no calcification could be detected.

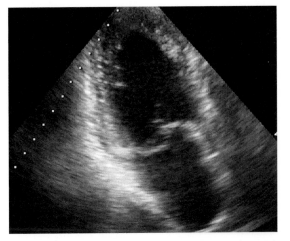

Prolapse of the posterior mitral leaflet is also visible in the apical two-chamber view.

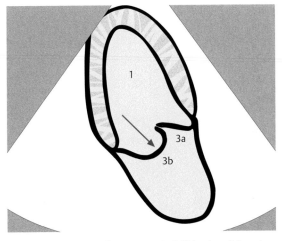

There is no typical thickening of the valve.

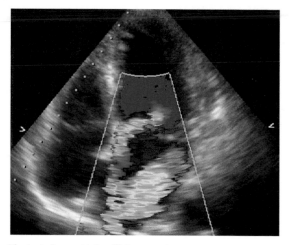

The typical eccentric insufficiency can be seen, ...

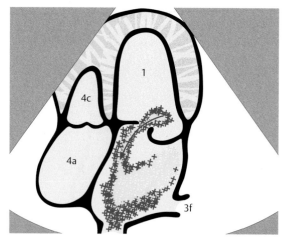

... which in myxomatous degeneration of the posterior leaflet usually points toward the atrial septum.

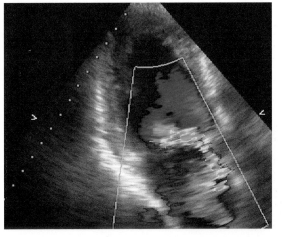

Mitral insufficiency should be displayed in several imaging planes ...

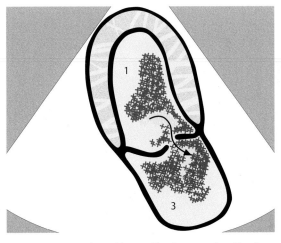

... to avoid overestimation or underestimation.

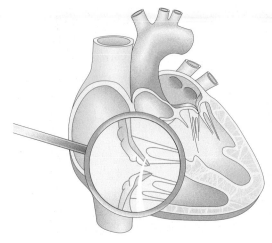

Degenerative changes in the tricuspid valve in tricuspid insufficiency.

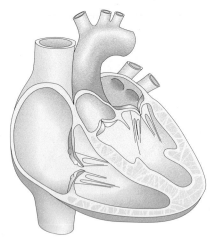

Retrograde flow across the tricuspid valve causes right heart dilatation.

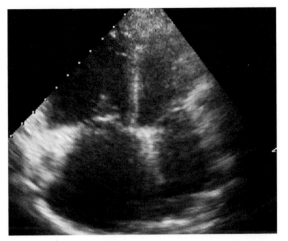

Right cardiac enlargement can be evaluated well in the apical four-chamber view.

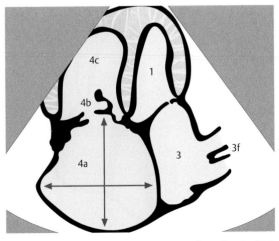

In this plane the right atrium can be measured in its longitudinal and transverse axes.

Cardiac Abnomalities

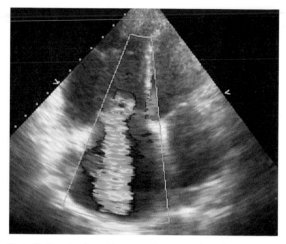

Typically there is a flamelike regurgitant jet in the right atrium.

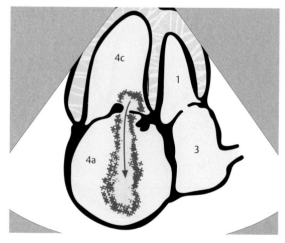

The extent of the jet can be used for quantification.

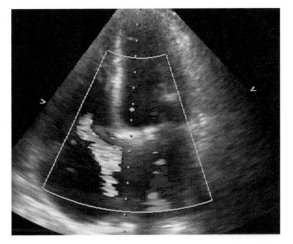

The regurgitant jet in tricuspid insufficiency is often directed eccentrically toward the atrial septum.

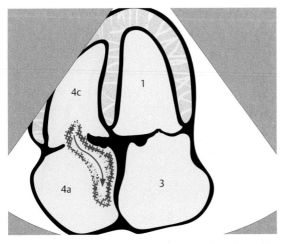

The regurgitant jet should be imaged in several planes if possible (apical four-chamber or five-chamber view, parasternal short-axis view).

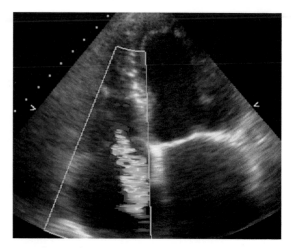

Minimal tricuspid regurgitation with a narrow-based regurgitant jet ...

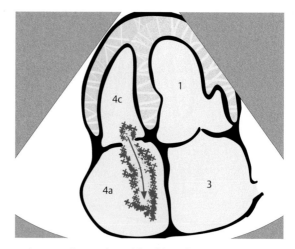

... almost reaching to the middle of the right atrium.

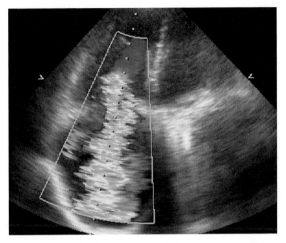

Severe tricuspid valve insufficiency results in a broader-based jet ...

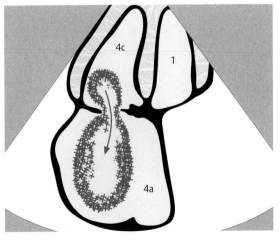

... filling more than half of the right atrium.

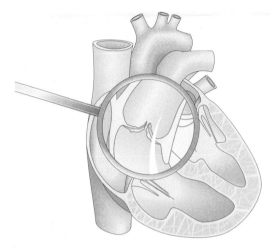

Degenerative valve changes in pulmonary insufficiency.

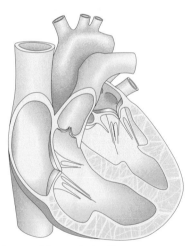

Volume overload causes right ventricular dilatation.

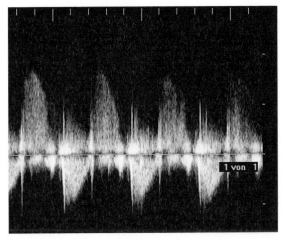

CW Doppler mode shows the regurgitant jet in the parasternal short-axis view.

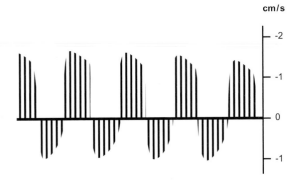

The recording shows the typical steplike diastolic signal, similar to aortic insufficiency.

Cardiac Abnomalities

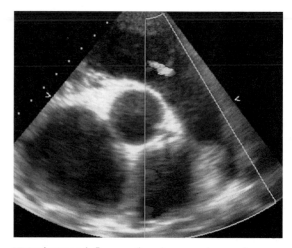

Minimal retrograde flow over the pulmonary valve can often be detected ...

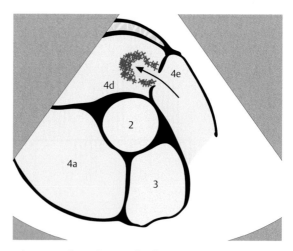

... but it is not hemodynamically relevant and does not involve risk of endocarditis.

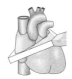

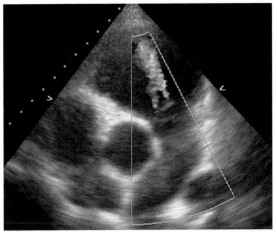

Notably greater retrograde flow across the pulmonary valve,
reaching to the middle of the right ventricle.

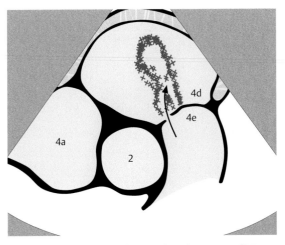

Given the "V" shape of the right ventricle, pulmonary insufficiency
can seldom be fully captured in just one plane.

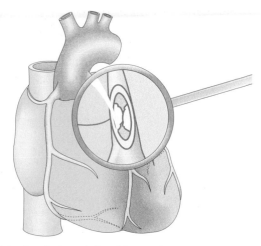

Anterior wall infarction due to occlusion of the anterior interventricular artery.

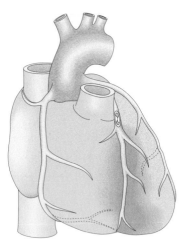

Segmental loss of contractility and thinning of affected myocardial areas related to scarring.

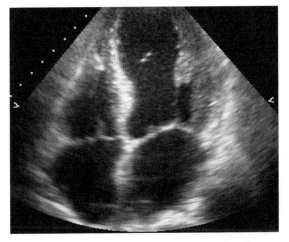

Impaired contractility can be imaged well in the apical windows ...

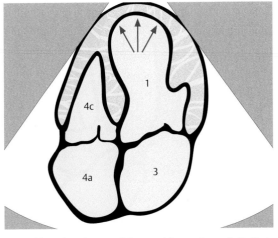

... although evaluation of the ventricle apex is usually limited.

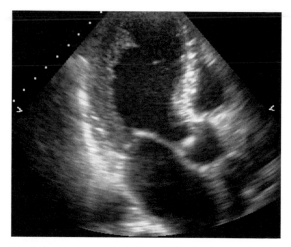

A typical consequence of anterior wall infarction is a saccular aneurysm ...

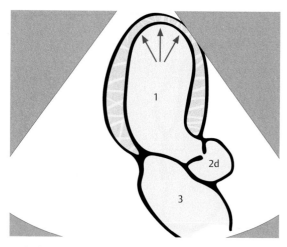

... which is preferably evaluated in an apical view.

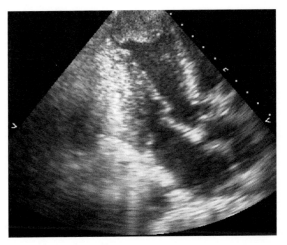

Especially in more recent infarctions, ventricular thrombi form over the infarcted ventricle segments ...

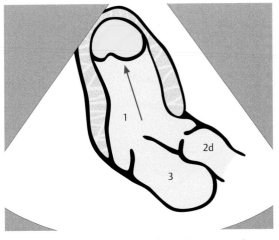

... appearing like a broad-based polyp in the aneurysmal areas.

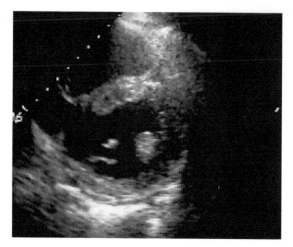

Infarction of the interventricular septum can lead to necrosis with a consecutive septal defect.

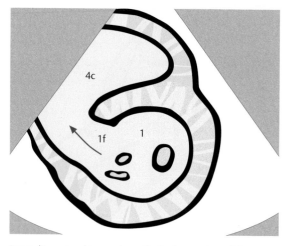

A two-dimensional image shows the broken contour of the interventricular septum.

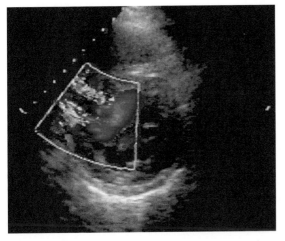

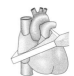

Color Doppler imaging shows overflow into the right ventricle ...

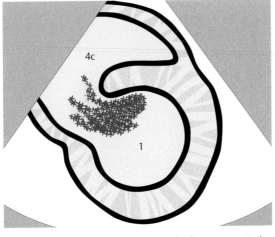

... and increased velocities as a result of various ventricular pressures.

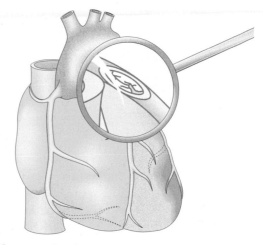

Myocardial infarction resulting from occlusion of the circumflex branch of left coronary artery ...

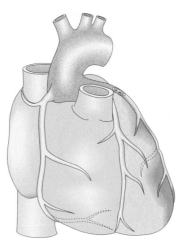

... with loss of contractility of the lateral wall.

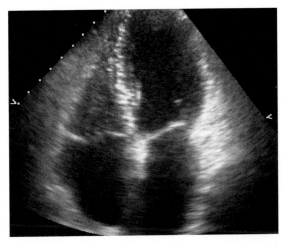

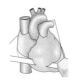

The akinetic ventricular segments can be seen in the apical four-chamber view.

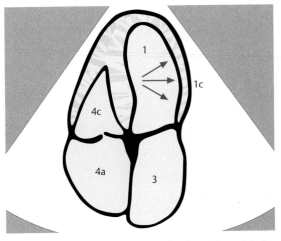

In less recent infarctions there is thinning of the ventricular musculature.

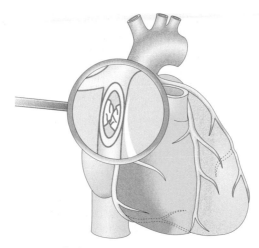

 Posterior wall infarction caused by occlusion of the right coronary artery.

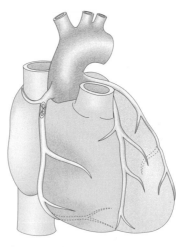

In right coronary dominance, the ventricular apex may be affected.

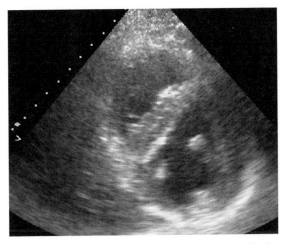
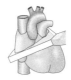

The akinetic posterior wall segments can be imaged in the parasternal short-axis view.

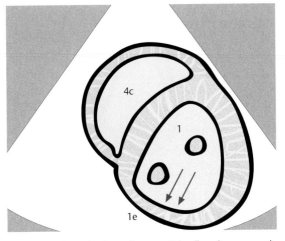

In this plane, the thinned myocardial wall can be measured.

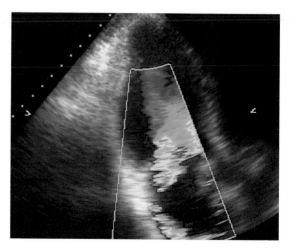

Larger infarctions involve the posteromedial papillary muscle, resulting in mitral insufficiency ...

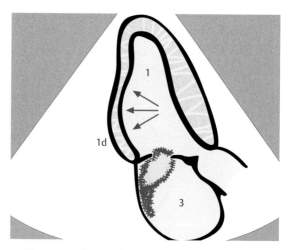

... with an eccentric regurgitant jet.

Cardiac Abnomalities

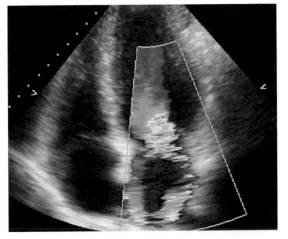

For more severe mitral insufficiency following posterior
wall infarction ...

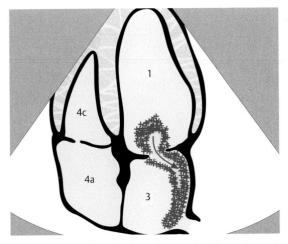

... a transesophageal echocardiogram should be performed
additionally to exclude rupture of the chordae tendinae.

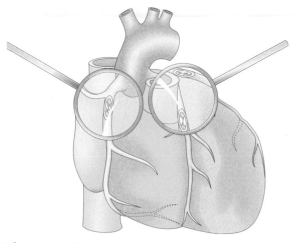

Infarction over a large surface area involving several myocardial areas is caused by diffuse occlusion processes ...

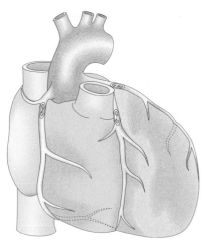

... and leads to dilatation of the left ventricle.

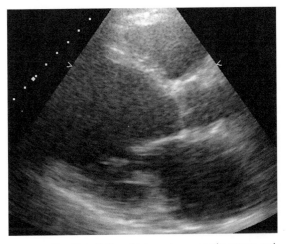

The dilated left ventricle can be seen in the parasternal long-axis view ...

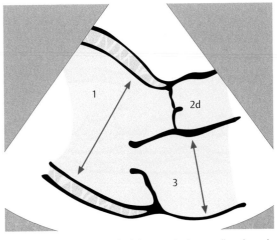

... whereby the left atrium is also usually enlarged.

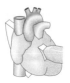

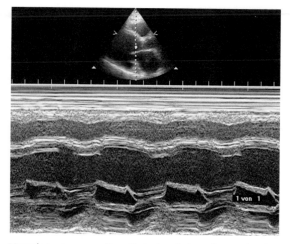

M-mode tracing across the mitral valve displays a low amplitude of mitral valve opening ...

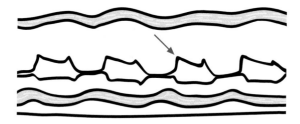

... thus indicating decreased transmitral inflow.

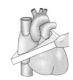

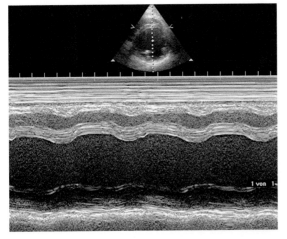

M-mode left ventricular tracing showing decreased contractility in systole ...

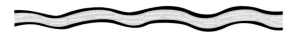

... as well as the increased diameter of the left ventricle.

Cardiac Abnormalities

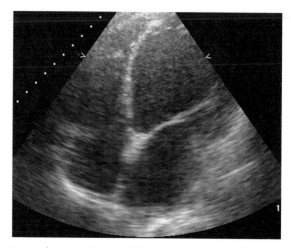

Ventricular contractions should be analyzed in the apical imaging planes ...

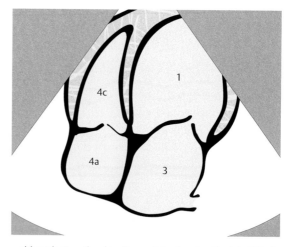

... although given the ubiquitous minimal contraction it is difficult to differentiate between infarcted and noninfarcted myocardium.

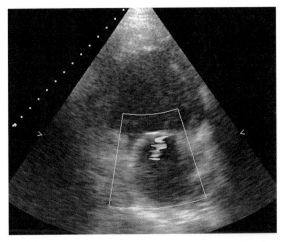

On account of left heart dilatation,
mitral insufficiency is observed ...

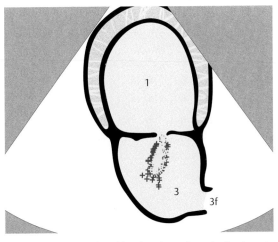

... although this is usually mild and not hemodynamically relevant.

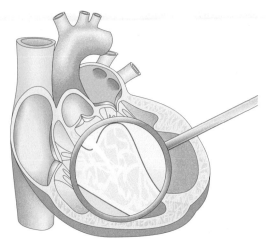

 Diffuse cardiomyopathy in dilated cardiomyopathy ...

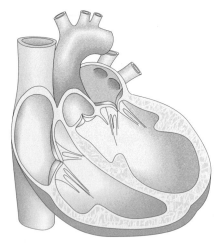

... with characteristic enlargement of all cardiac cavities.

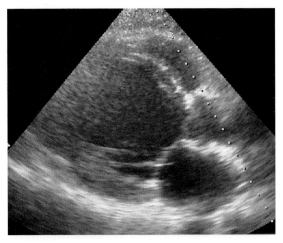

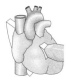

The diameters of the dilated left ventricle and the left atrium are preferably evaluated in the parasternal long-axis view.

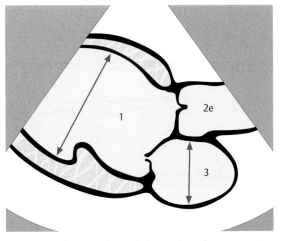

Impaired contractility, and often tachycardia, is noticeable.

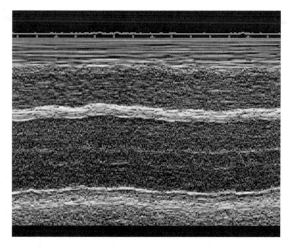

M-mode tracing can evaluate systolic and diastolic diameters of the left ventricle.

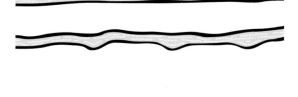

Impaired left ventricular function can be demonstrated on account of the almost failing systolic contractions.

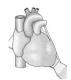

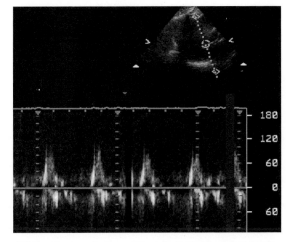

PW Doppler recording across the mitral valve shows tachycardia
and reduced flow velocities ...

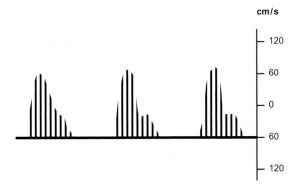

... as a sign of decreased stroke volume.

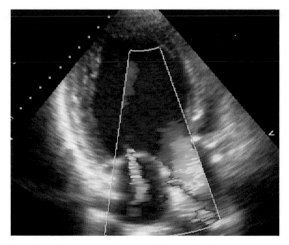

Dilatation often enables detection of (relative) mitral insufficiency ...

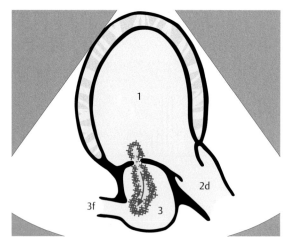

... which is usually only minimal. If mitral insufficiency is more severe, an additional transesophageal examination is advisable.

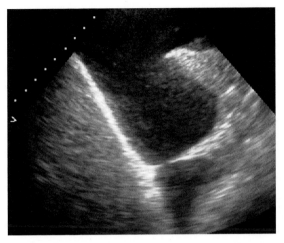

Pleural effusion can develop due to abnormal pump function.

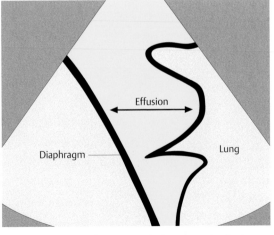

Effusions can be seen by orienting the beam past the diaphragm
in the posterior axillary line (patient in the supine position).

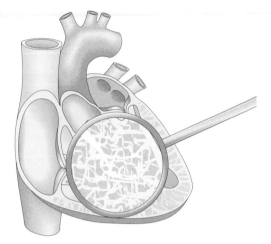

Isolated hypertrophy near the interventricular septum ...

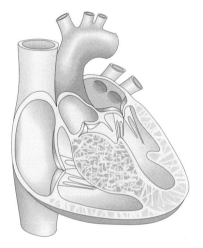

... with impairment of systolic outflow from the left cardiac chamber.

Cardiac Abnomalities

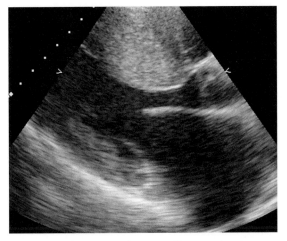

In the parasternal view septal hypertrophy appears ...

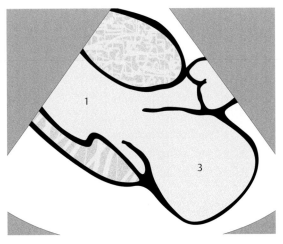

... as a balloonlike swelling.

Cardiac Abnomalities

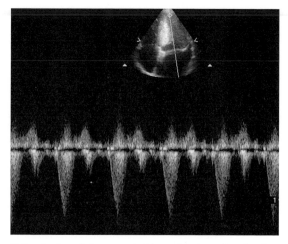

CW tracing is made from an apical three-chamber or five-chamber view in the outflow tract of the left ventricle.

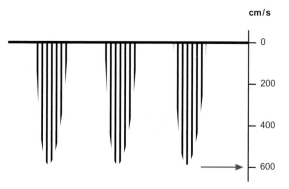

A V-shaped gradient demonstrates the obstruction to the outflow tract.

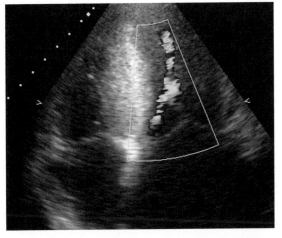
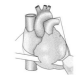

The change in color seen in color Doppler imaging indicates hypertrophy of the septum and increased infundibular flow velocity.

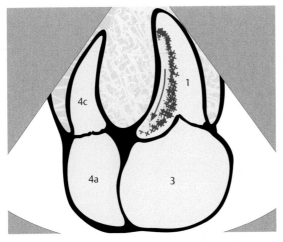

CW tracing is the modality of choice for quantification (pressure gradient at rest or after provocation).

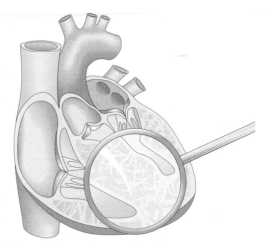

Abnormal thickening of the musculature involves all ventricular areas ...

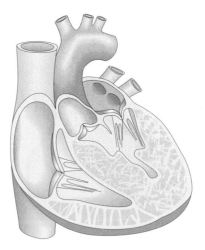

... and leads to a reduction in the size of the ventricular cavity.

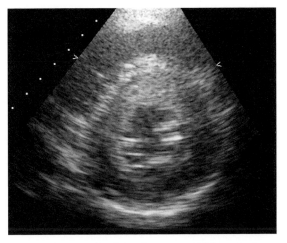

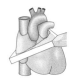

A cross-sectional view shows symmetric hypertrophy ...

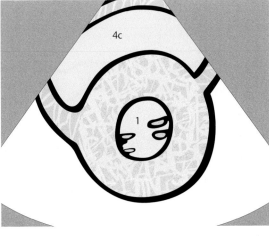

... with just minimal remaining volume in the left ventricle.

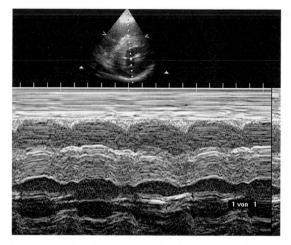

M-mode recording shows hypertrophy of the anterior and posterior walls with ...

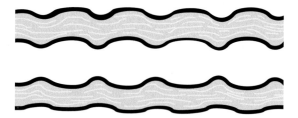

... reduced systolic amplitude of contraction.

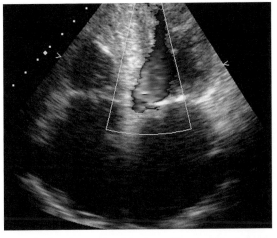
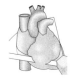

Color Doppler imaging did not reveal increased flow velocity in systole ...

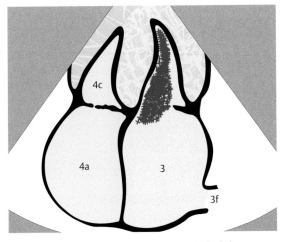

... and thus implied a lack of obstruction.

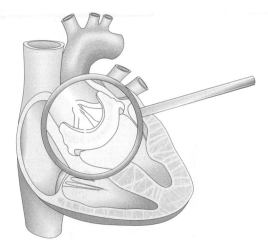

Bioprosthetic valves comprise a suture ring with struts, upon which pericardium or porcine aortic valves are mounted.

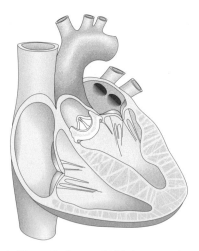

A residual effect of the aortic disease which led to surgical intervention is postoperative left ventricular hypertrophy which regresses with time.

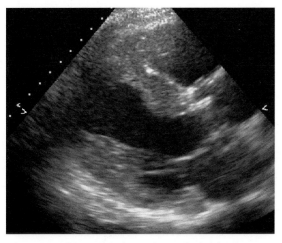

The annulus of the bioprosthetic valve is only slightly echogenic.

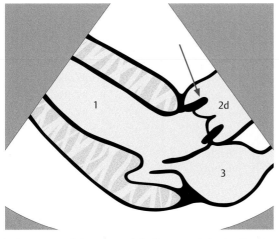

In the parasternal view, the aortic leaflets can only be visualized to a limited extent.

Cardiac Abnormalities

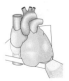

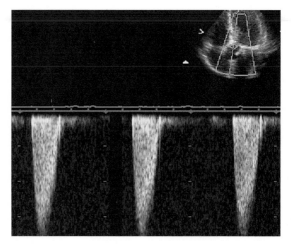

CW Doppler imaging showing the U-shaped flow profile ...

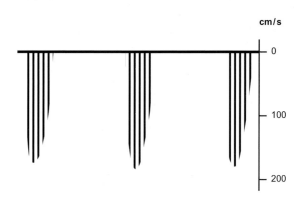

... which is identical to that of a native aortic valve.

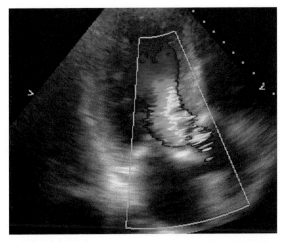

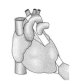

Color Doppler imaging can show increased flow velocity across the valve ...

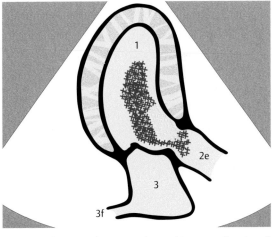

... however, this is seen often and is not usually a sign of degeneration.

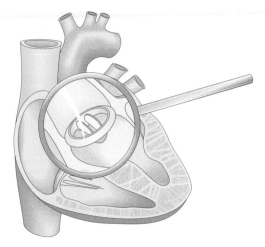

▶ Commonly used artificial prostheses consist of a suture ring and a bileaflet prosthetic valve.

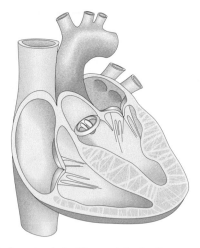

▶ Left-ventricular hypertrophy is still present shortly after surgery, but it usually regresses with time.

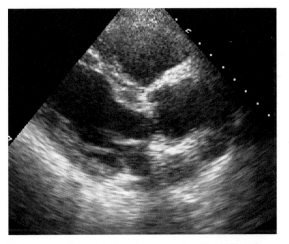

The parasternal long-axis view shows reverberation artifacts from the valve leaflets.

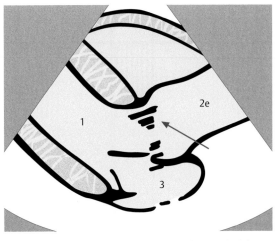

Individual valvular structures can barely be distinguished due to reverberation artifacts.

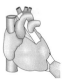

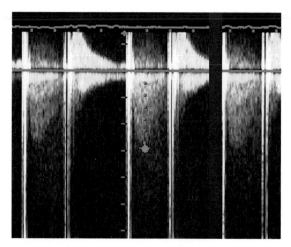

At the beginning and end of systole, typical clicks caused by the artificial leaflets appear in transaortic CW Doppler.

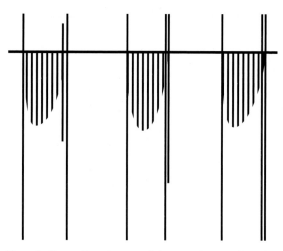

Flow velocity over the valve normally increases to approximately 2 m/s, depending on valve type and size.

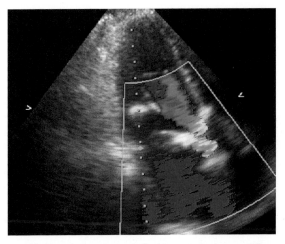

Color Doppler imaging typically demonstrates increased flow velocity.

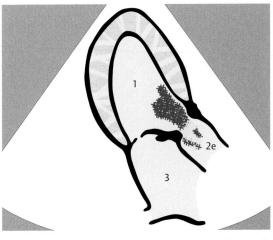

This is not considered pathological.

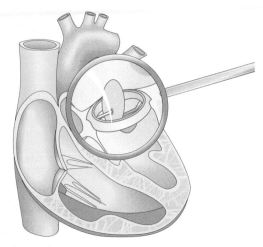

Commonly used artificial prosthetic valves in the mitral position consist of a sutured ring and a tilting-disk valve.

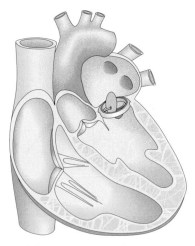

Left atrial dilatation is frequent and is considered to be a sign of prior left atrial overload from the mitral valve defect.

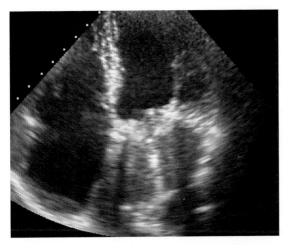

Considerable echo artifacts from artificial valves complicate the
evaluation of individual cardiac structures.

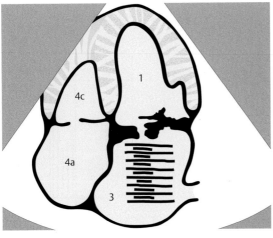

Especially in the apical views, the left atrium can be barely
visualized.

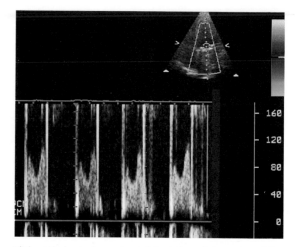

Clicks at the beginning and end of diastole mark the motion of the disk-valve prosthesis.

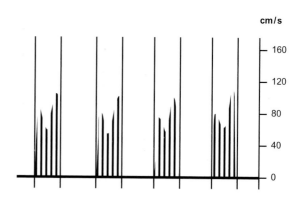

The CW Doppler image shows the typical mitral inflow profile and thus regular valve function.

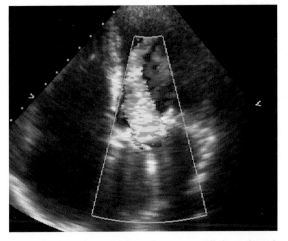

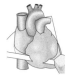

Inflow over the artificial prosthesis can usually be evaluated adequately with color Doppler imaging. However, the left atrium cannot be visualized.

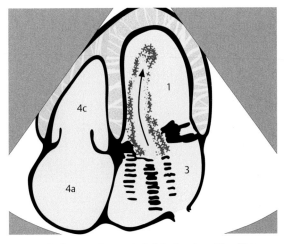

In the case of suspected clinically relevant insufficiency, a transesophageal echocardiogram should be performed.

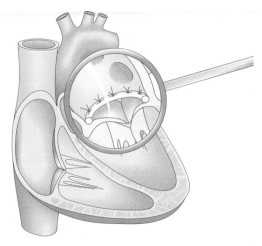

Insufficient leaflets can be reinforced by suturing an artificial ring in the valve annulus.

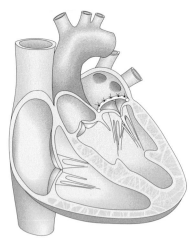

Often there is also left atrial dilatation and possibly also signs of right heart overload.

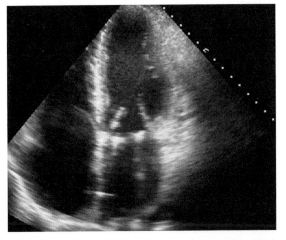
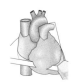

The ring is imaged as an echodense area near the base of the mitral valve ...

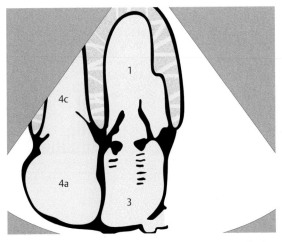

... and can easily be mistaken for sclerosis of the native mitral valve annulus.

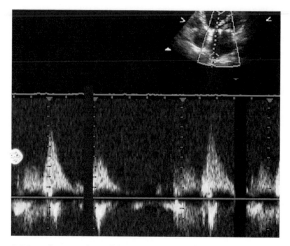

CW Doppler recording of the mitral valve from an apical location shows regular inflow in the left ventricle without any sign of stenosis.

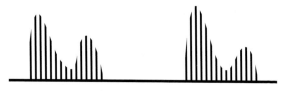

Insufficiency may also be recorded, but should be diagnosed using color Doppler imaging.

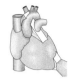

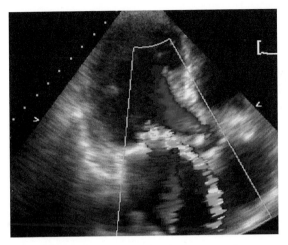

Color Doppler imaging can reveal residual insufficiency ...

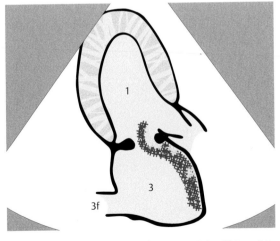

... with an eccentric insufficiency jet.

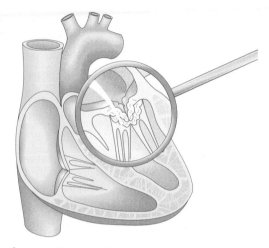

Inflammatory changes in the mitral valve with typical vegetations on the valve edges.

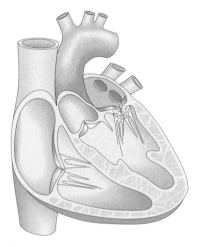

Resulting mitral insufficiency can lead to left atrial dilatation and right heart enlargement.

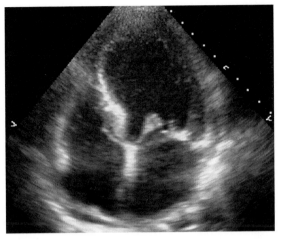
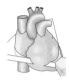

Endocarditis vegetations with polypoid coatings ...

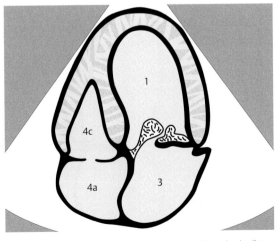

... mostly on the free edges of the valve leaflets.

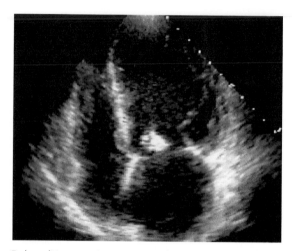

Endocarditis vegetations can cause echodensities as well as calcification ...

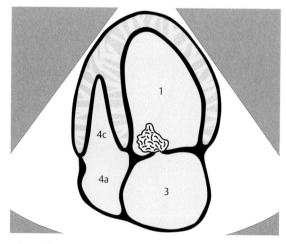

... but still be highly mobile.

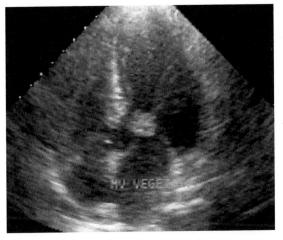

Polyplike vegetations ...

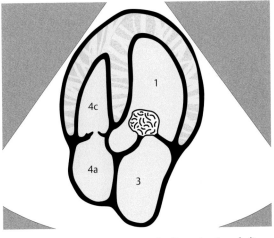

... can lead to systemic embolism.

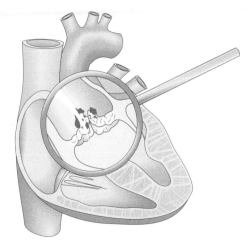

Especially in previously damaged leaflets, complicating endocarditis can occur.

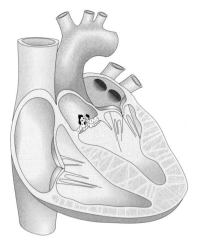

As in the mitral valve, the free edges of the valve leaflets are often affected.

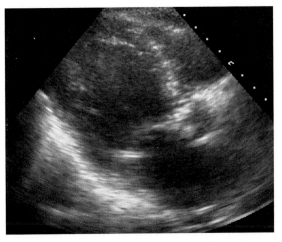

The aortic leaflets should be examined in all planes ...

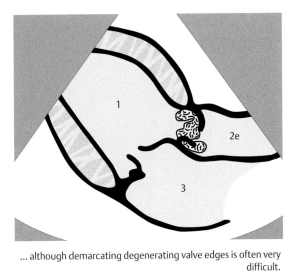

... although demarcating degenerating valve edges is often very difficult.

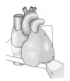

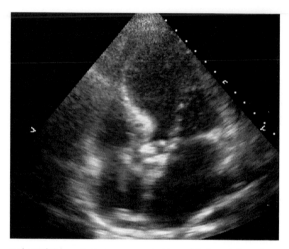

Endocarditis vegetations are remarkably mobile in systole and diastole ...

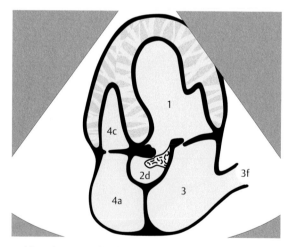

... although compared with mitral valve endocarditis they are less noticeable given the smaller valve leaflets.

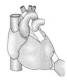

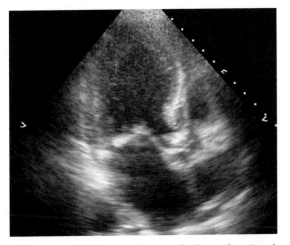

In case of a presumptive diagnosis, both transthoracic and transesophageal echocardiography should be repeatedly performed ...

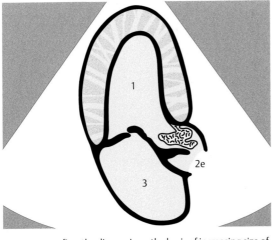

... to confirm the diagnosis on the basis of increasing size of vegetations.

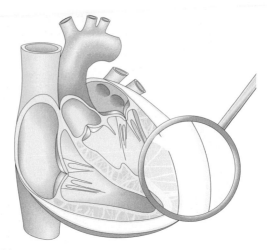

 Separation of the pericardium due to effusion.

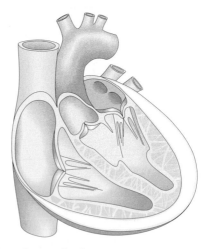

If effusion is hemodynamically relevant, ventricular compression occurs.

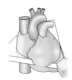

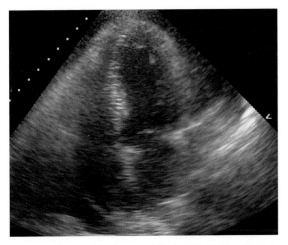

Extensive effusion, especially chronic effusion, does not necessarily cause hemodynamic impairment.

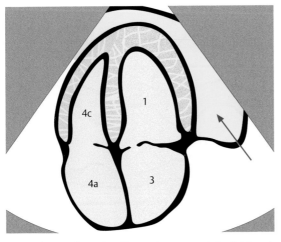

The two-dimensional image shows normal-sized atria and ventricles. Functional effectiveness should not be assumed, however.

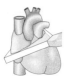

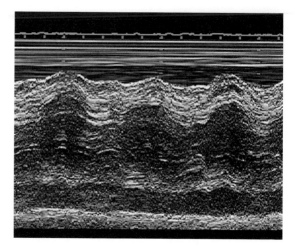

In hemodynamically irrelevant pericardial effusion, ventricular diameter is normal ...

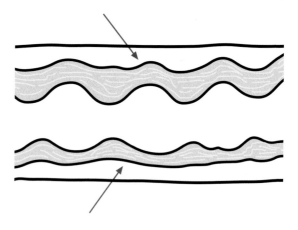

... as is systolic contraction.

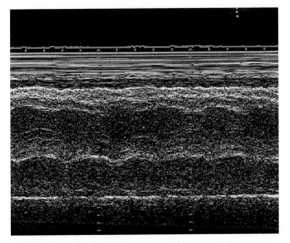

Tamponade resulting from pericardial effusion typically involves tachycardia and reduced ventricular diameter ...

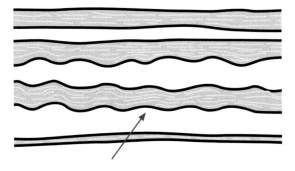

... as well as limited systolic contraction due to impaired inflow.

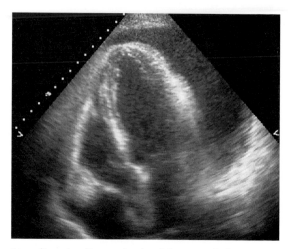

A two-dimensional image of pericardial tamponade shows compromised ventricles ...

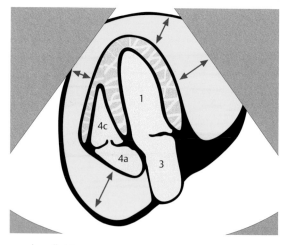

... and small atria.

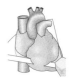

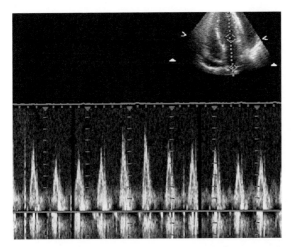

Typically, there is pronounced respiratory fluctuation of
intracardiac flows (here transmitral inflow) ...

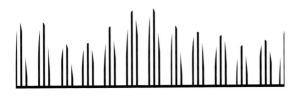

... due to the varying filling volume and stroke volume depending
on the respiratory phase.

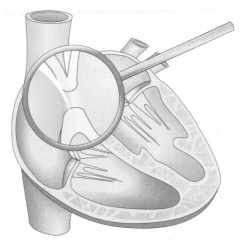

Primary defect in the atrial septum in atrial septal defect (ASD) II.

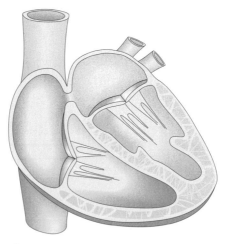

There is usually a left–right shunt which leads to right heart enlargement.

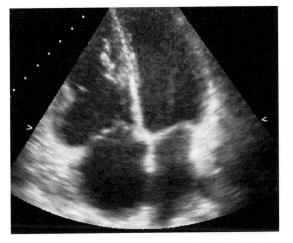

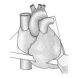

The markedly enlarged right heart shown in the two-dimensional image is typical for atrial septal defects.

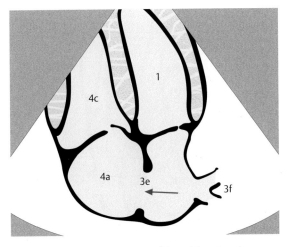

Inadequate imaging of the atrial septum, however, is not evidence, as it is reflected inadequately in apical views.

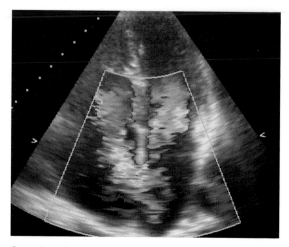

If transthoracic visualization is good, the left–right shunt can be clearly imaged.

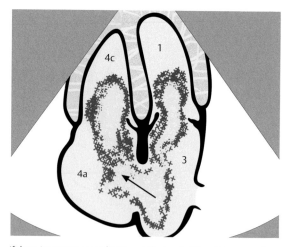

If there is pressure equalization at the level of the atrium as well as limited visualization, the transthoracic examination is insufficient to exclude ASD.

**Cardiac Abnomalities**

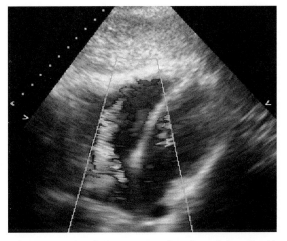

If there is suspicion of ASD, imaging in the subcostal plane should also be attempted ...

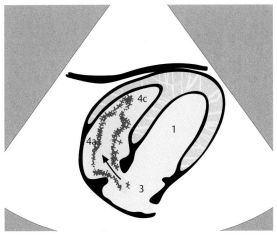

... because the shunt flow in this view is sharply angulated toward the transducer and thus can be better recorded.

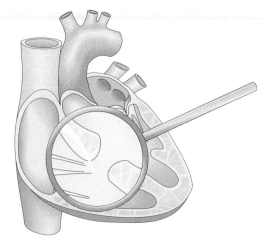

Ventricular septal defects can vary in terms of size and localization.

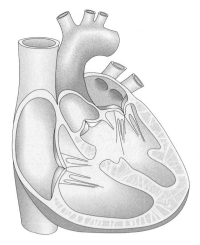

In smaller defects only the left–right shunt is detectable; larger defects involve left ventricular dilatation.

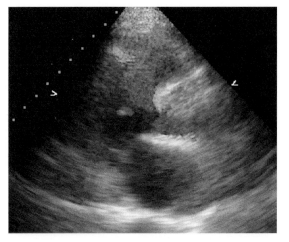

Two-dimensional imaging can sufficiently reveal the broken contour of the ventricular septum ...

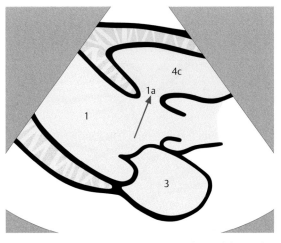

... in larger defects only.

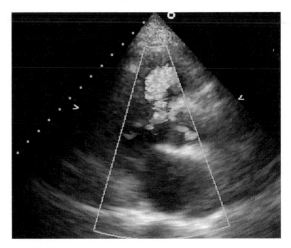

Shunt flow is displayed as a darting flamelike increase in flow velocity in the right ventricle ...

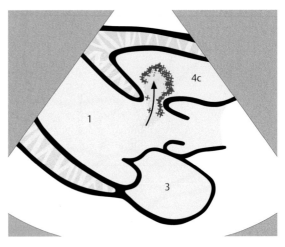

... which can be readily seen in the parasternal view.

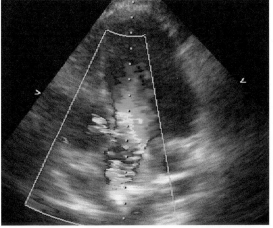

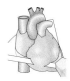

Shunt flow cannot be imaged as well in apical views ...

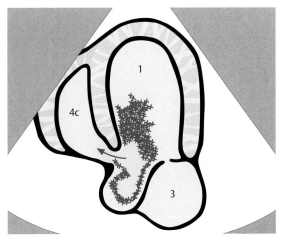

... because it runs at a right angle to the axis of the ultrasound beam.

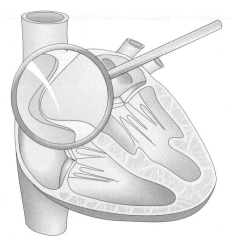

 Saccular aneurysm of the atrial septum.

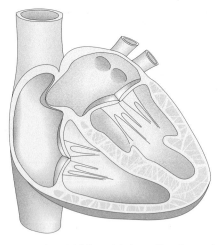

If there is a concurrent septal defect, right heart dilatation results from the left–right shunt.

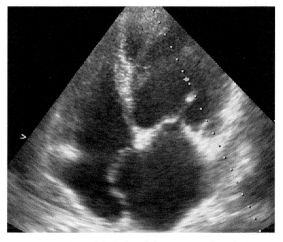

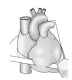

Typical deviation of the aneurysmal atrial septum.

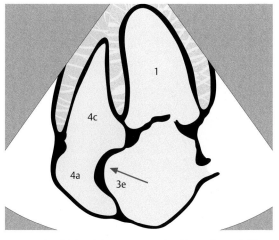

An atrial septal aneurysm can lead to cardiac embolism.
Transesophageal echocardiography can detect adherent thrombi.

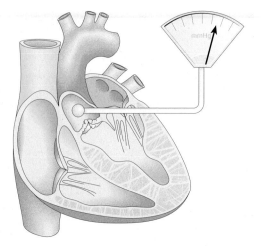

Pressure overload in the systemic circulation causes secondary changes ...

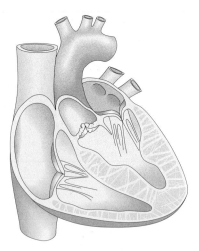

... such as left ventricular hypertrophy and aortic valve sclerosis.

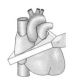

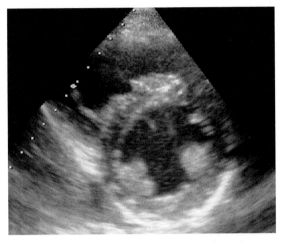

Thickening of the left ventricular walls can be seen.

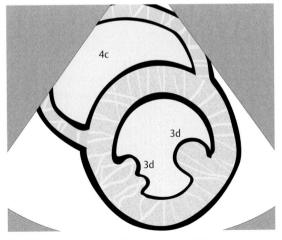

For surveillance check-ups, left ventricular wall thicknesses, as well as end-systolic and end-diastolic diameter, should be recorded.

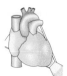

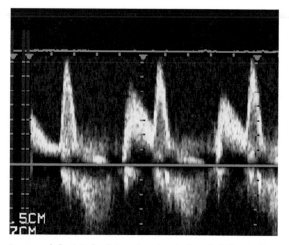

Decreased elasticity leads to reduced early diastolic inflow in the left ventricle.

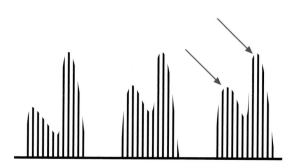

The inverse profile of transmitral inflow is considered evidence of diastolic dysfunction.

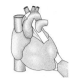

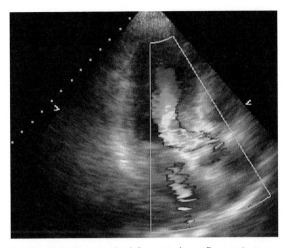

In infundibular hypertrophy, left ventricular outflow can increase over the septum as well as ...

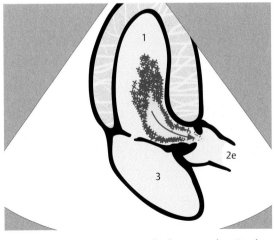

... across the degenerated aortic valve.

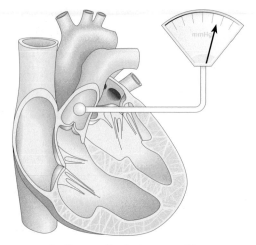

Right cardiac pressure overload is caused by displacement of the pulmonary artery flow tract as well as left cardiac disease.

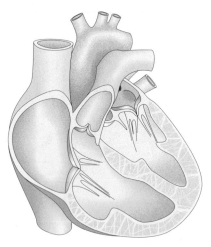

Under conditions of longstanding increased pressure, the right heart is dilated and the right ventricle hypertrophied.

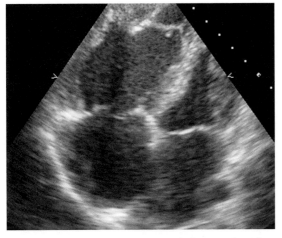

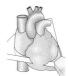

Pronounced right ventricular hypertrophy with ...

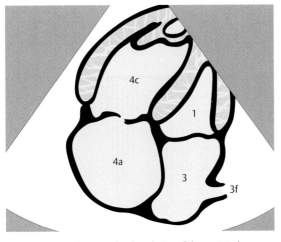

... increased trabeculation of the ventricular apex.

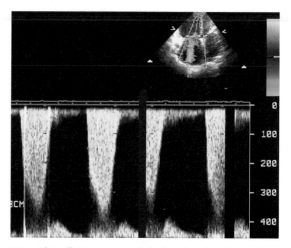

Tricuspid insufficiency can usually be found resulting from right cardiac dilatation and increased pressure.

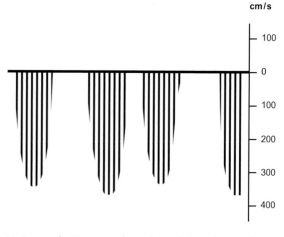

Maximum velocities are used to estimate right cardiac apical pressure.

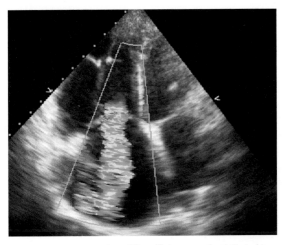

Concomitant tricuspid insufficiency can be detected in a four-chamber view.

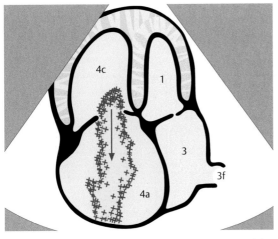

Surveillance check-ups should describe the extent of the regurgitant jet.

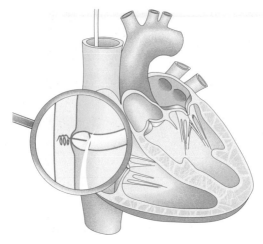

AAI pacemaker in the right atrium.

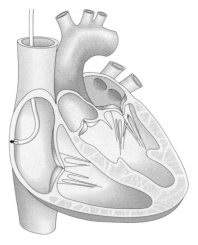

The pacemaker lead is positioned in a J-shape on the right lateral atrial wall.

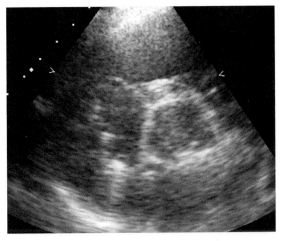

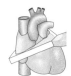

The metal wire leads cause considerable artifacts.

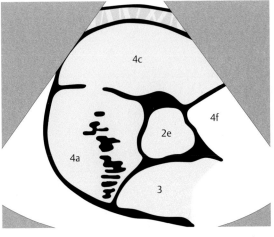

The path of the wire is thus difficult to visualize.

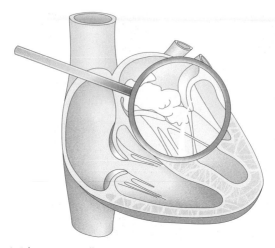

 Atrial myxoma usually originates in the septum ...

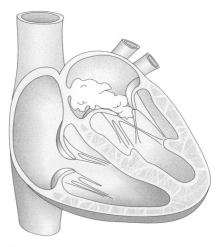

... and has a villous surface.

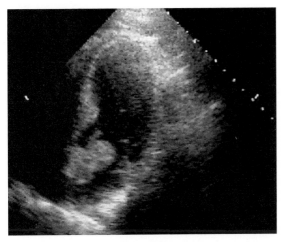

Larger myxomas can protrude into the mitral valve in diastole.

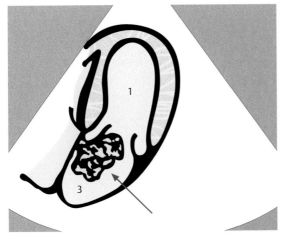

On the one hand they can obstruct inflow into the left ventricle and on the other hand they can cause systemic embolization.

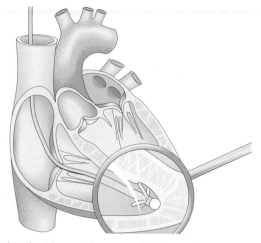

Pacemaker leads in the right ventricle are typically placed in the apex.

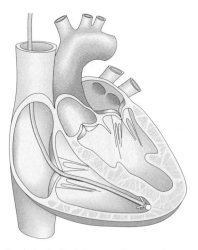

The electrical stimulation in the right ventricle causes deformation of the ventricular complex in a fashion similar to left bundle branch block.

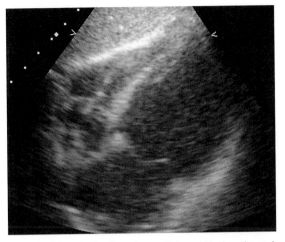

The elongated path can be readily imaged in the subcostal window.

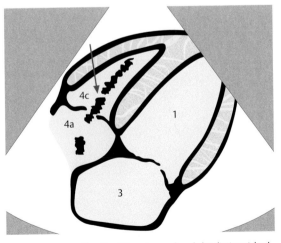

The tip of the wire can barely be distinguished.

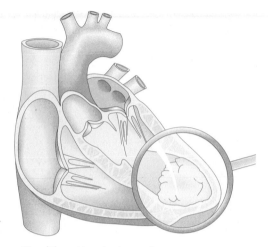

Sometimes appositional thrombi can be detected in anterior wall aneurysms ...

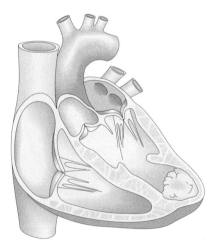

... which can cause cardiac embolism.

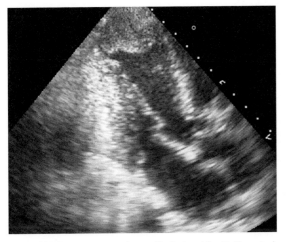

Sacculated aneurysms can be readily distinguished in the apical imaging planes.

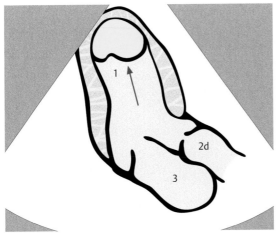

The thrombus is broad-based and sessile, demonstrating a homogeneous reverberation pattern.

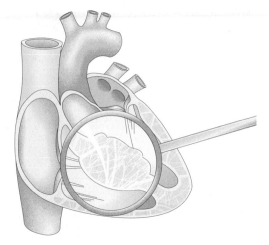

Malignant primary ventricular tumors are usually mesenchymal in origin.

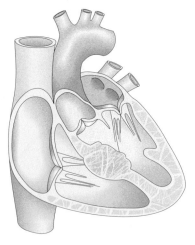

The most commonly occurring are angiomyosarcoma and rhabdomyosarcoma.

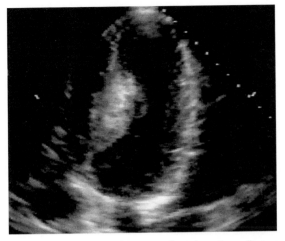

The ventricular septum shows irregular swelling ...

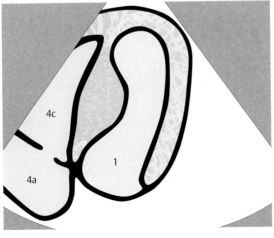

... and can cause functional intraventricular obstruction.

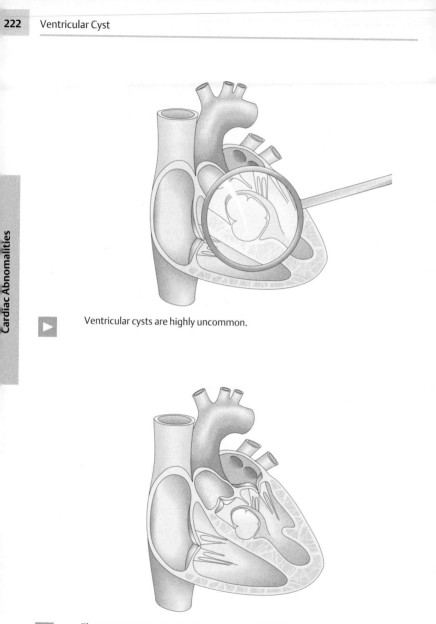

Ventricular cysts are highly uncommon.

They can cause marked electrocardiographic (EKG) changes.

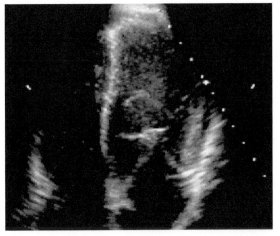

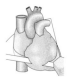

The cyst wall can be readily distinguished in an apical view.

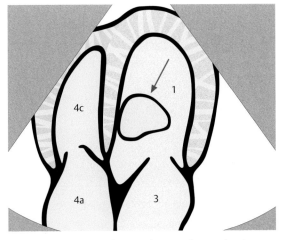

Color Doppler imaging does not show any flows within the cyst.

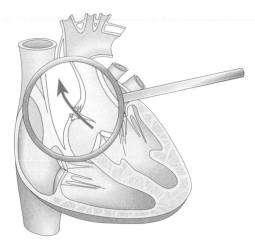

Dissecting aortic aneurysms arise from separation of the intima from the media ...

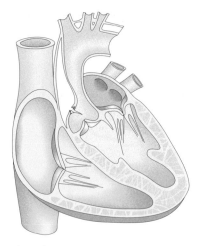

... and can extend into the supra-aortic arteries or abdominal aorta.

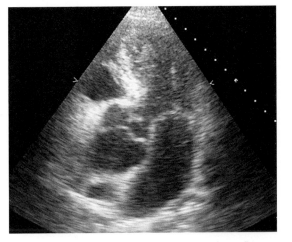

The separated intima can be seen as an echodense, floating
membrane ...

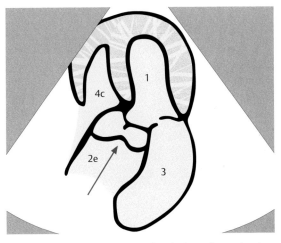

... directly above the aortic valve.